Contemporary Topics in Patient Safety - Volume 1

Edited by Stanislaw P. Stawicki and Michael S. Firstenberg

Published in London, United Kingdom

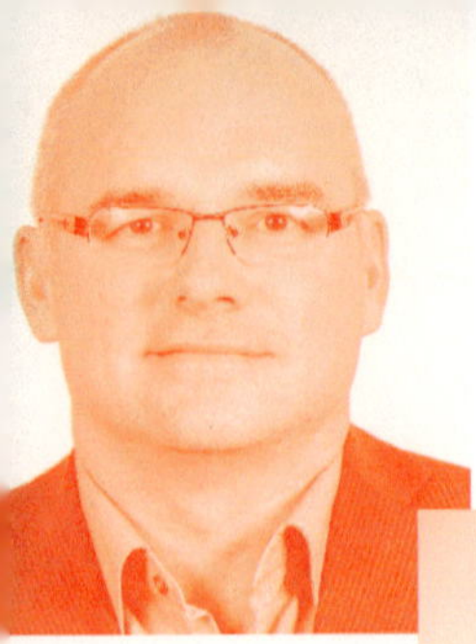
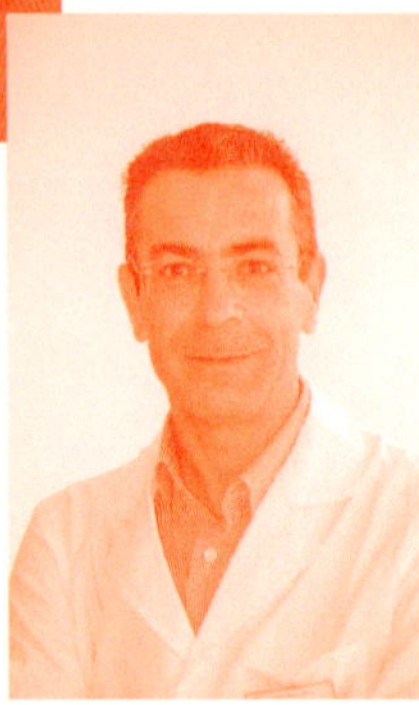
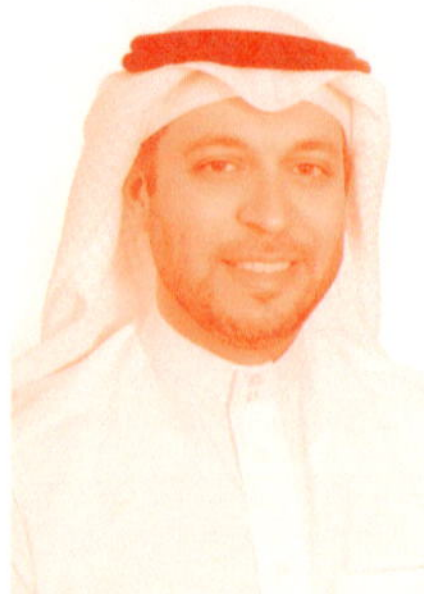
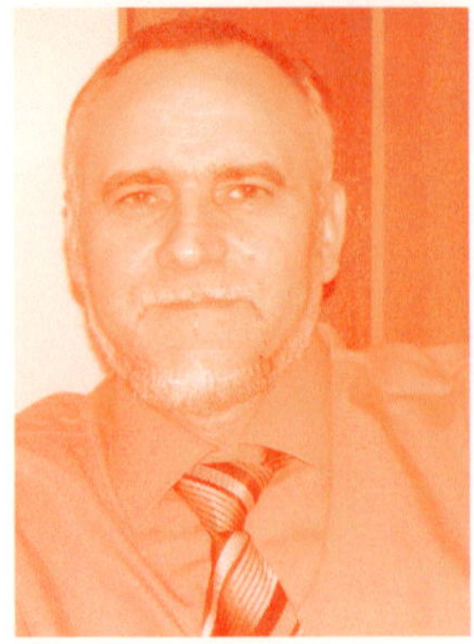
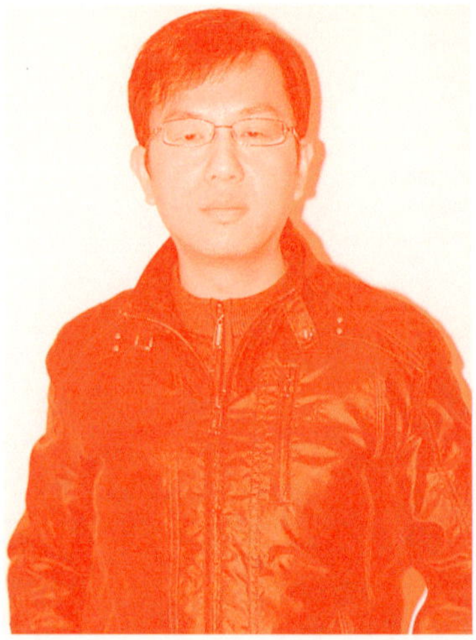
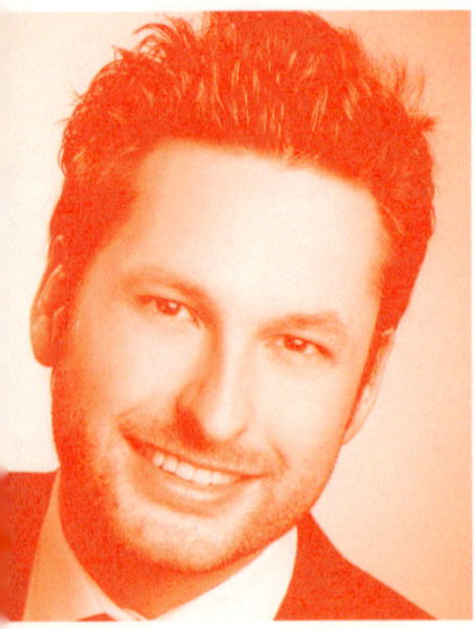
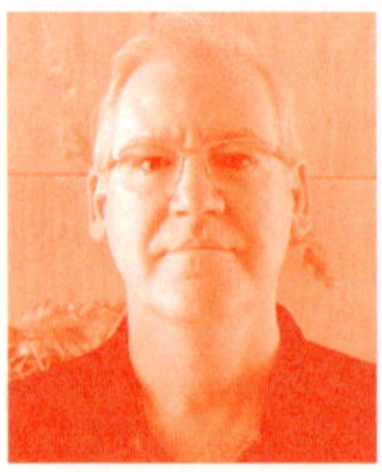

IntechOpen

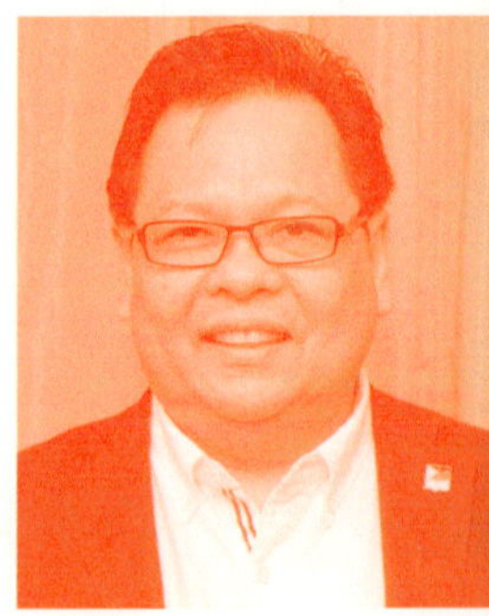
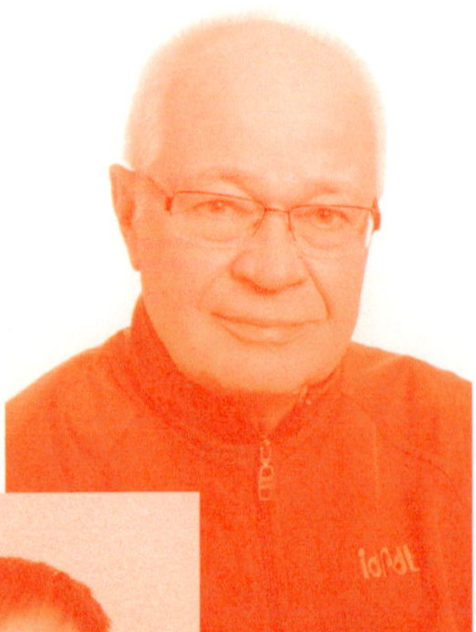
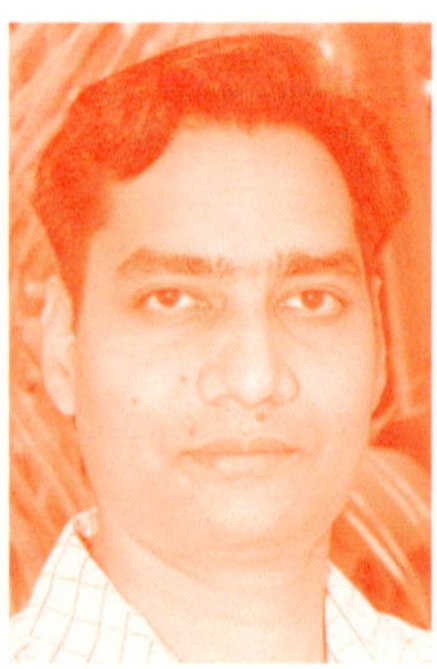
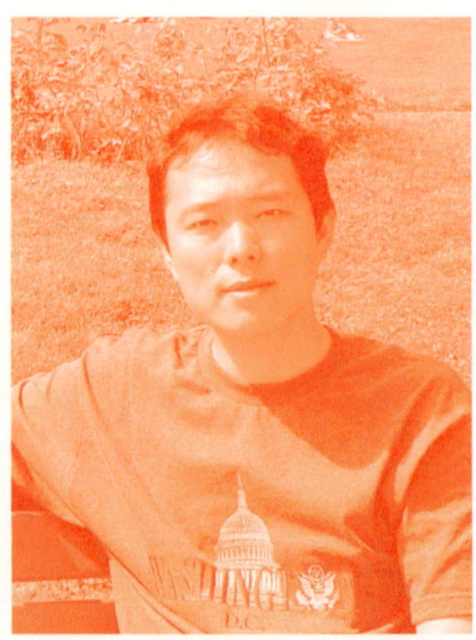
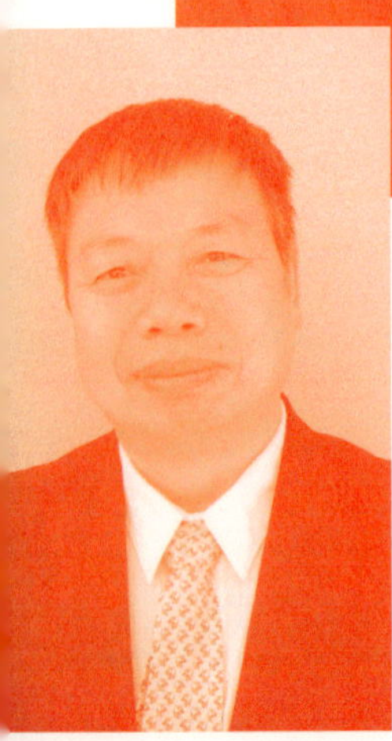
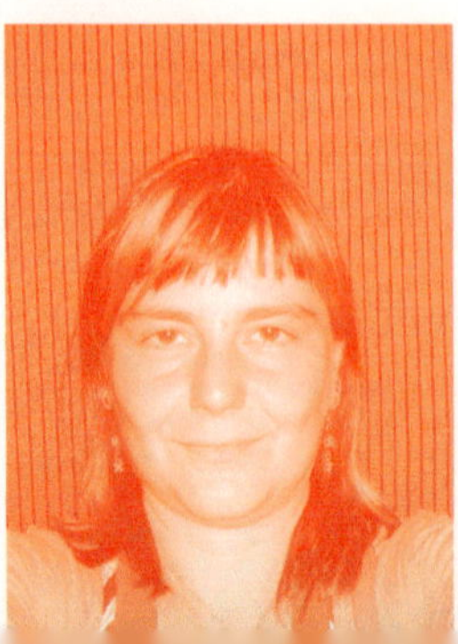

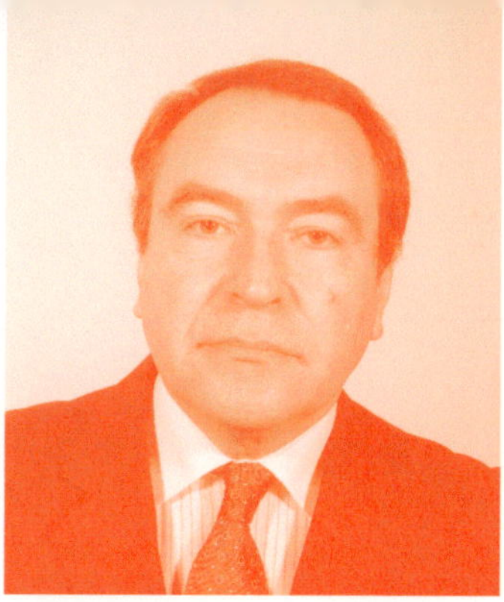
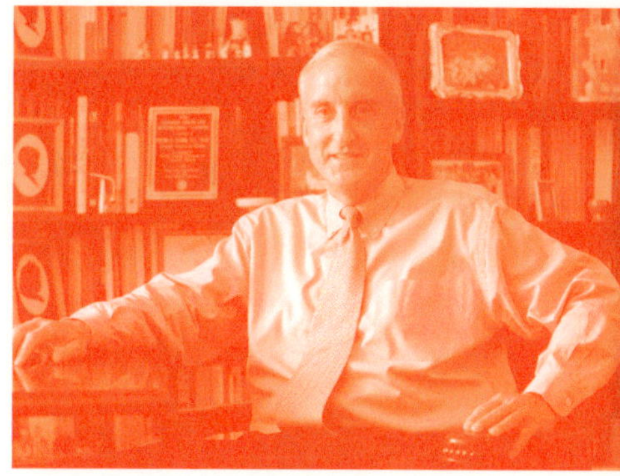
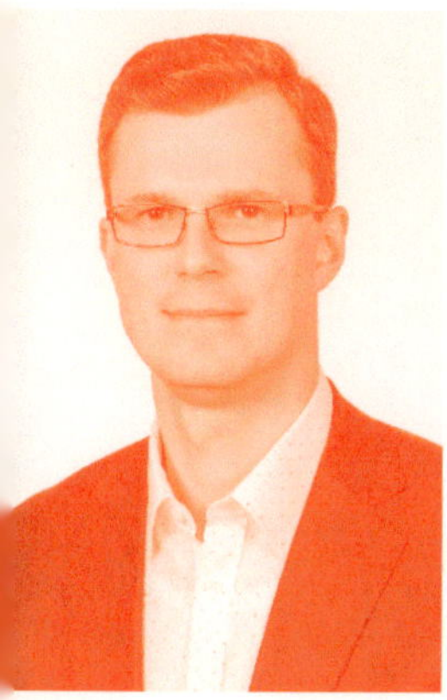
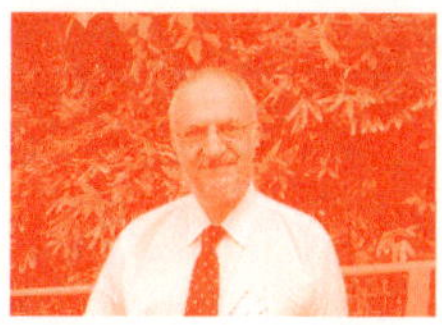
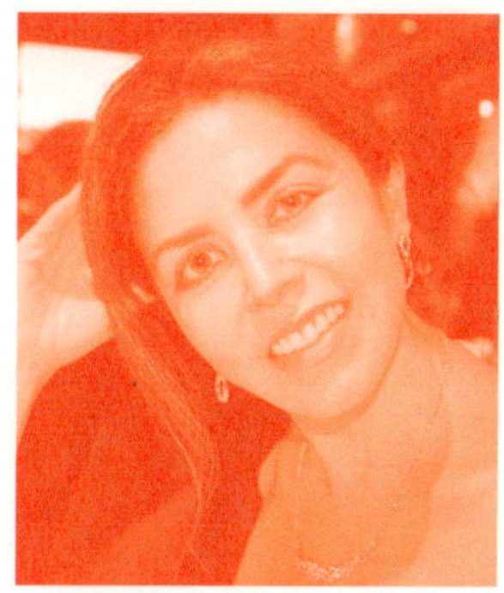

Supporting open minds since 2005

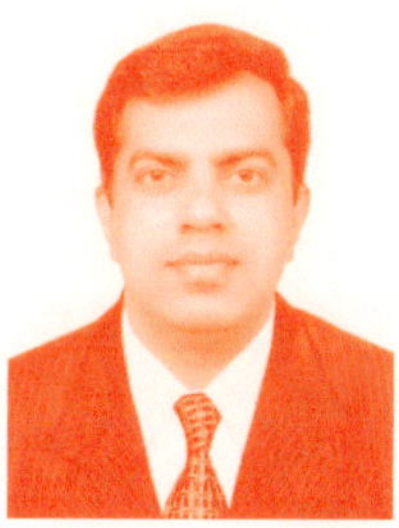
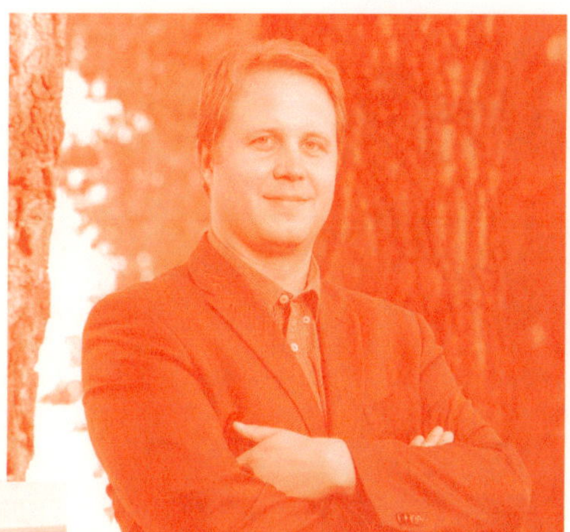
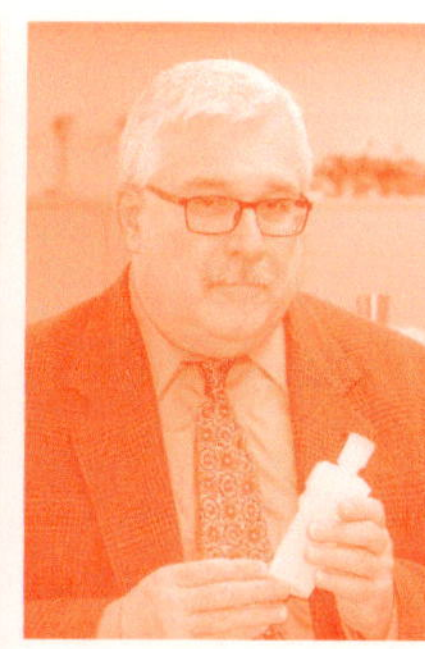
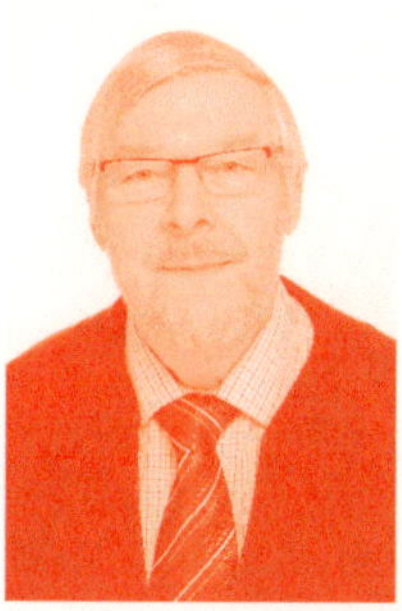
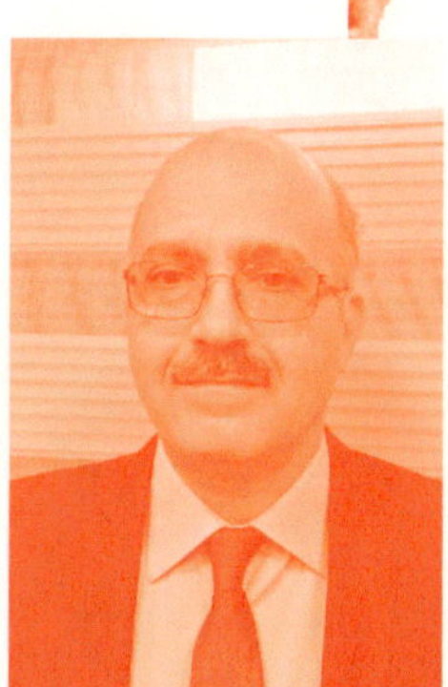
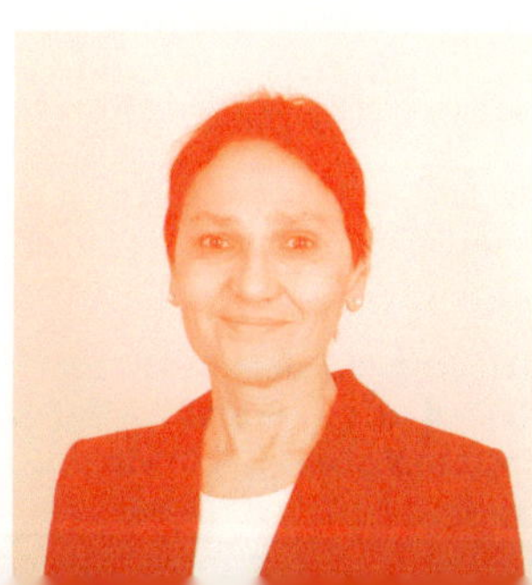
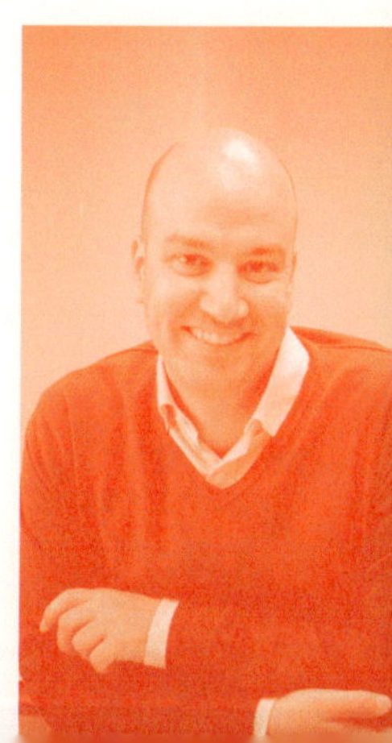

Contemporary Topics in Patient Safety - Volume 1
http://dx.doi.org/10.5772/intechopen.87616
Edited by Stanislaw P. Stawicki and Michael S. Firstenberg

Contributors
Sule Biyik Bayram, Nurcan Çalişkan, María Desamparados Bernat Adell, Ana Folch Ayora, María Sánchez Galán, Pablo Salas Molina, Eladio Joaquín Collado Boira, Ahmed Umar Otokiti, Pratyusha Gaonkar, Hoda Sabati, Amin Mohsenzadeh, Nooshin Khelghati, Myra van den Goor, Tanya Bondarouk, Thomas L. Logan Morgan, Sandy Konerth, Gregory Domer, Thomas M. Gallagher, Shekiba Shahabzada, Juliana Sotherland, Elisabeth N. Paul, Kushee-Nidhi Kumar, Bryan Wilson, Shilpa Salpekar, Parampreet Kaur, Stanislaw P. Stawicki, Michael S. Firstenberg, James P. Orlando

First published in London, United Kingdom, 2022 by IntechOpen
IntechOpen is the global imprint of INTECHOPEN LIMITED, registered in England and Wales, registration number: 11086078, 5 Princes Gate Court, London, SW7 2QJ, United Kingdom
Printed in Croatia

British Library Cataloguing-in-Publication Data
A catalogue record for this book is available from the British Library

Additional hard and PDF copies can be obtained from orders@intechopen.com

Contemporary Topics in Patient Safety - Volume 1
Edited by Stanislaw P. Stawicki and Michael S. Firstenberg
p. cm.
Print ISBN 978-1-83962-403-2
Online ISBN 978-1-83962-404-9
eBook (PDF) ISBN 978-1-83962-405-6

For EU product safety concerns:
IN TECH d.o.o., Prolaz Marije Krucifikse Kozulić 3, 51000 Rijeka, Croatia, info@intechopen.com or visit our website at intechopen.com.

Meet the editors

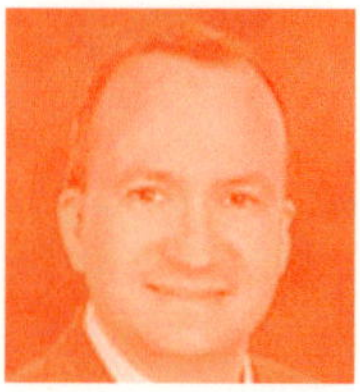

Dr. Stawicki is a Professor of Surgery and Chair of the Department of Research & Innovation, St Luke's University Health Network, Bethlehem, Pennsylvania. A specialist in general surgery and surgical critical care, he has co-authored nearly 700 scholarly works, including more than 20 edited books. In addition to national and international medical leadership roles, Dr. Stawicki is a member of numerous editorial boards. His areas of expertise include blockchain technology, patient safety, academic leadership, mentorship, trauma/critical care, and sonography.

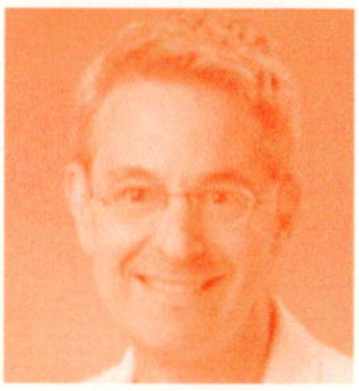

Dr. Michael S. Firstenberg is a thoracic surgeon at the St. Elizabeth Medical Center (Ascension), Appleton, Wisconsin. He attended Case Western Reserve University Medical School, Cleveland, Ohio, received his general surgery training at University Hospitals in Cleveland, and completed thoracic surgery fellowships at The Ohio State University and The Cleveland Clinic. He is an active member of the Society of Thoracic Surgeons (STS), American Association of Thoracic Surgeons (AATS), American College of Cardiology (ACC), and American College of Academic International Medicine (ACAIM), for which he served as president in 2021–2022. He has authored more than 250 peer-reviewed manuscripts, abstracts, and book chapters and has edited several textbooks and lectured worldwide on topics ranging from medical leadership, COVID-19, endocarditis, and extra-corporeal membrane oxygenation (ECMO).

Contents

Preface

This volume is the fifth in our book series dedicated to patient safety. As this collection of chapters and books evolved over the years, it has become clear that despite the tremendous amount of global enthusiasm regarding the topic of patient safety, the ultimate goal of "zero harm" may be just about as remote today as it had been a decade ago. That said, we must continue to strive for better outcomes, improved quality, and enhanced safety, and although it may seem that these constant efforts are taking us to an unreachable ending, the gravity and importance of what is at stake make this approach "the only way to go." Without a doubt, when we explore the broader area of patient safety, we need to understand and define all the conceptual elements involved within the overall framework of modern healthcare. Furthermore, it is also imperative that we make every attempt to understand the consequences – and not just to the patient being treated who is at risk for an unsafe event or encounter – but all aspects of the healthcare system from the individual providers to the system as a whole, including the potential global impacts.

At this point, it is well recognized that adverse events, or broadly understood and defined "harm," play a significant role in the outcomes of patients as they journey through the healthcare system. Defining such events can be challenging, regardless of whether done in real-time or retrospectively. From a most basic standpoint, such patient safety events can be viewed as an undesirable consequence of a healthcare process or procedure that is performed or implemented during a patient's hospital course, or in fact during any healthcare encounter, no matter how mundane in character. While classic high-profile examples may include events such as medication errors, catheter-related infections, falls, wrong-site surgery, and communication or handoff breakdowns, it is important to recognize that such harm can also occur as a result of failures to act, failures to recognize/rescue, competency gaps, educational deficits, delays in care secondary to process or system (or staffing) challenges, and even (as the global healthcare community is seeing more and more of during the coronavirus disease 2019 [COVID-19] pandemic) limitations to timely and appropriate access to healthcare due to limited resources and/or overwhelmed system capacity.

While it is easy to appreciate that when "harm" – or broadly understood breakdown in patient safety – occurs the impact is greatest on the patient and their families, at the same time, it also must be recognized that such events can have much broader implications. Without a doubt, when adverse events happen to patients, regardless of the magnitude, they can result in potential pain and suffering, but also significant increases in costs to the health care system. Even though various studies attempted to estimate the financial implications of breakdowns in safety, the overall math is somewhat unclear with regards to the costs of lost quality or productive of life, increased need for testing or subsequent care, prolonged hospitalizations, and the impact on resources available to devote to other patients – especially in those environments in which there are substantial limits on the ability to provide comprehensive and unrestricted care to all.

Over time, patient safety events adversely affect the wider well-being of a community and society, with consequences that can be appreciated on many levels. Breakdowns in patient safety can also have dramatic impacts on the healthcare team. It is well established that provider burnout is a growing concern. While burnout can be attributed to a variety of factors, the personal and professional accountabilities or sense of "failure" can result in a significant emotional toll, especially on those directly involved in caring for patients. At times, providers may feel inadequate, powerless, or hopeless when directly involved in safety breakdowns while providing care. Even though "everyone wants what is best for the patient," this concept can reflect a continuum of engagement, support, or enthusiasm especially when care is dependent on a high-functioning and engaged multidisciplinary team in which roles and responsibilities can often be poorly defined. Lapses in patient safety can have a variety of negative consequences on the entire team, especially when such lapses are perceived to be potentially preventable. At the same time, under strong leadership, high-performance institutional culture, and empowered teams, tremendous individual and team satisfaction can be derived from objective progress and improvements in patient safety. This, in turn, can contribute significantly to a personally and professionally gratifying and healthy organizational milieu. After all, "a rising tide lifts all boats" with regard to successful patient safety initiatives motivating and empowering a team.

A cornerstone to establishing a culture focused on improving patient safety, as discussed throughout this book series, is that a paradigm shift must take place, with the transition away from placing blame on an individual or even a process or system breakdown, and increasingly toward exploring such events as opportunities to understand "how and why" such patient safety issues evolve and develop. This modern approach is much more effective in helping to objectively improve and sustainably strengthen our healthcare systems. While there are clearly events that ultimately are the result of single individual actions (or inactions), improvements can only come when there is a broader understanding of why such events occur and what mechanisms are in place to prevent or mitigate them under the umbrella of assumption of innocence, goodwill, and fully acknowledging that no one is perfect. While individual educational and competency issues might (and often do) impact specific events, initiatives must be in place to not only address the individual using a reasonable and timely peer-review process but also, even more importantly, explore the much broader topic of why such gaps exist and what practical and reasonable approach can be proposed to address them. Except for very rare circumstances, removing or limiting an individual from participation in a healthcare team should not be considered the best or first-line tactic. Such topics must be explored proactively and continuously, and if there are recurrent themes or patterns of concern, a team-based approach – as reviewed extensively in these volumes – should be the first-line approach to addressing any issues identified in the process.

When this book project started, we focused on a vignette-based format to help the authors tell a story in a matter in which readers can better understand and appreciate the potential real-life implications of the challenges faced and the benefits of searching for a solution. In this volume, we transition to a concept-based discussion. The two approaches are complementary, and when combined serve to increase the understanding of longitudinal and multi-disciplinary cause-effect relationships that is critical to developing effective and durable patient safety initiatives. We also acknowledge and emphasize with each new volume that the concept of patient safety, or the reduction of harm, does not imply that harm is likely to be eliminated completely. Rather, it is our goal to provide various tools to help minimize any potential risks to a patient as much as possible. Unfortunately, as the cumulative body of patient safety literature grows, some of which is addressed in the current book, it becomes evident that initiatives focused on improving patient safety are not without unintended consequences and/or secondary harm. As such, as we all continue on this journey, we need to recognize that any initiative to improve patient care by reducing risk and the potential for harm also requires continued monitoring to not only ensure the desired goals are met but also that unintended consequences are appropriately addressed and managed in a timely manner.

The editors wish to extend their unconditional appreciation to all of those involved in bringing this project to completion. Not only do we want to thank all the authors who dedicated significant time and effort to writing and refining their chapters, but we also want to acknowledge the staff of IntechOpen who provided tremendous support, motivation, and encouragement during the publication process. We also want to extend gratitude to our families, friends, and colleagues for their understanding and patience in response to the countless hours of work required to complete this ambitious project. We are immensely grateful for the opportunities to raise the level of awareness of patient safety and related issues among our truly global readership.

Stanislaw P. Stawicki
Department of Research and Innovation,
St. Luke's University Health Network,
Bethlehem, Pennsylvania, USA

Michael S. Firstenberg
Department of Cardiothoracic Surgery,
St. Elizabeth Medical Center,
Appleton, Wisconsin, USA

Chapter 1

Introductory Chapter: Patient Safety and Quality of Care - Inextricably Linked and Absolutely Essential Components of Modern Healthcare

James P. Orlando, Michael S. Firstenberg and Stanislaw P. Stawicki

"Those who cannot remember the past are condemned to repeat it."
- George Santayana.

1. Introduction

Modern healthcare is characterized by two dominant forces—constant change and increasing complexity [1]. The emergence of this modern paradigm dates to approximately 20–30 years ago when the distressing awareness of the system-wide impact of medical errors on patient outcomes and healthcare costs came into focus [2, 3]. With this realization came another revelation—that human performance, team dynamics, communication, and systems-based practice require significant modifications to achieve safety, quality, and performance records that even remotely approximate those of the air transportation, nuclear energy, banking/finance, or other high-reliability industries [2, 4].

The current book initiative reflects a much-needed new addition to our series entitled *Vignettes in Patient Safety*. When the overall project started several years ago, the focus was to allow authors to contribute their thoughts and experiences based on a clinical vignette, whether actual or hypothetical. The opportunities that these chapter contributors saw to improve on the safety and efficiency of delivering healthcare in a very complex and multidisciplinary environment were highlighted. What quickly became evident through the extensive diversity of submissions was the global recognition of how challenging it is to provide high-quality, safe patient care. Even the most simple of problems often required very challenging solutions, with frequently unexpected and/or unpredictable outcomes. Part of the challenges identified in our earlier endeavors included the vast diversity of systems, processes, multidisciplinary teams, and individuals that must come together to achieve a common goal. Even in the best of circumstances the motivations, incentives, and agendas can be quite divergent, and while consensus building is often required, it becomes imperative that the primary goals (and thus the overarching agenda of patient safety) remain intact.

IntechOpen

2. Patient safety reflects quality and value

The relationship between high quality services, patient safety, and the resultant added value is becoming increasingly evident with the growing complexity of our healthcare systems. Within this general context, we must note that good patient outcomes are a result of high quality care delivered by competent and highly trained professionals, at the right time, for the right reasons, and with impeccable care and precision [5, 6]. Given the above considerations, it is not surprising that healthcare institutions that focus on patient safety and care quality are emerging as leaders, and not only doing so in the short-run, but more importantly, in a long-term, sustainable fashion. Key organizational characteristics that correlate with better and safer patient care include the encouragement of in-house quality and safety initiatives, where effective "positive feedback loops" are created that continually reinforce high performance levels and system-based learning and improvement [7]. It is also very important to note that the best system can only be as strong as its weakest link. Consequently, broadly administered educational and training efforts that focus on patient safety and care quality are required at organizational level. Part of this new educational paradigm is the assurance that critical knowledge is not only communicated but also retained, applied, and periodically reinforced.

3. The importance of patient safety education

When transitioning from general educational considerations to more focused, provider-centric initiatives, we must emphasize certain key emerging concepts regarding healthcare provider training and its impact on both care quality and patient safety. Does it matter where a resident completes their training? We know that choosing a post-graduate residency or fellowship is one of the most important decisions medical students will make in their career. Interestingly, there have been several studies and data insights that suggest their decision about where to apply and train for residency may carry consequences that go well beyond what was originally understood. The reason why it may be a "higher stakes" decision is because the various impacts of the imprinting of skills, techniques, attitudes, and behaviors that one gains during residency in the long-term perspective, especially, as it ultimately affects the physician's practice and their patients' outcomes. As several studies point out, physicians practice "how they were trained" and thus, where they trained and for how long, most certainly affects multiple downstream manifestations of their post-graduate training and future clinical performance [8–10].

Further examination of the published literature also suggests that if residents train in learning environments with high quality outcomes, then they will tend to practice in the manner that produced those high-quality outcomes when working as an independent attending. For example, in their 2009 paper on evaluating obstetrical residency programs using patient outcomes, Asch, et al., found that obstetrics and gynecology training programs can be ranked by the maternal complication rates of their graduates' patients [9]. The authors conducted a retrospective analysis of all Florida and New York obstetrical hospital discharges between 1992 and 2007 and connected those discharges back to physicians and their training programs. Furthermore, researchers at the Dartmouth Atlas Project, a group that uses Medicare and Medicaid data to analyze healthcare outcomes in national, regional, and local markets, has observed that "Physicians who train at institutions with better, more patient-centered, and efficient care will be better prepared to lead the transformation of health care when they are in practice" [11]. Collectively, the above studies and data insights seem to pass the "validation-test" with colleagues as well. Hospitals and health systems with high-quality outcomes have a strong cultural focus on patient safety and their patient safety education programs. These organizations are what Carroll and Rudolph described in their 2006 paper on how to design high-reliability healthcare organizations [12]. The takeaway is that patient safety education has not only a short-term impact on direct bedside care but a long-term impact on safety and outcomes as well. Given this new understanding we can readily see just how important it is where a resident trains.

4. Safety systems and patient safety champions

While it can be argued that there has been tremendous improvement in patient safety initiatives at all levels within our increasingly complex healthcare system, it must also be recognized that there are always opportunities for improvement. The concept of accepting "average performance only" results in a slippery slope of complacency and an individual or system-wide tolerance toward faults that ultimately may contribute to harm. Even though it is difficult, if not impossible, to directly attribute a single defect within any complex system or process, it must be recognized that "opportunities for harm" evolve over time and ultimately contribute to what is considered the "Swiss cheese model" of patient harm [2, 13]. Rarely does a single "opportunity" in the continuum of patient care result in an adverse or catastrophic outcome. Rather, unsafe systems are characterized by a series of "overlooked opportunities" over time, usually present during the course of the patient's healthcare encounter.

It has long been known that the avoidance of patient harm requires the constant presence of adequate and proactive oversight. Such oversight cannot be facilitated by a single individual or even a small group of highly committed individuals—there are simply too many "moving parts" for a small group to be effective. Rather, systems considered to possess excellent quality and safety records are characterized by the development of ubiquitous patient safety champions [14]. Within this progressive new framework, patient safety and care quality appear to be directly proportional to the omnipresence of patient safety champions, throughout the entire organization, and within each critical patient care process. Accountability is mutual, and non-judgmental feedback creates the sense of "common mission."

At the same time, top organizational leadership must actively support and develop patient safety champions, and unless key stakeholders sufficiently value this tremendous amount of work, energy, resources, and are ready to commit financial (and other) obligations that are required to effectively invest in patient safety, it becomes difficult for even the smallest of initiatives to gain traction. Furthermore, while it is difficult to draw a direct correlation between the investment in patient care initiatives and objective outcomes at times, such activities must be ingrained in the culture of an institution and viewed in a positive light. Even though objective outcomes in patient care initiatives can be somewhat challenging to demonstrate, their importance cannot be understated. Therefore, pertinent metrics and expectations should be defined in advance before any further steps are undertaken.

5. The patient safety journey

The patient safety journey outlined in this collection of chapters touches on many important points that are directly relevant to everyday clinical practice and systems-based healthcare operations. From a focus on teams to simulation to electronic health records utilization, the content included herein stresses the importance of constructive and synergistic approaches toward ensuring the provision of quality and safety our patients deserve. Similarly, the various chapters in this volume explore the importance of concepts as diverse as multi-disciplinary approaches, camaraderie, and simulation, to help attain the most important singular and ultimate goal—a "zero defect" healthcare environment [13, 15]. One key aspect, unique about the current book - and we would like to heavily stress this - is the increased emphasis on the critical importance of training on patient safety and care quality during the graduate medical education phase of professional development. That said, we also emphasize that patient safety and care quality, as inseparable components of the healthcare value equation, constitute a life-long journey for each and every individual involved in caring for, and ensuring the well-being of, another human being.

Within the above context, it is critical to recognize that simply "going through the steps" to "check a box"—although certainly a good start—does not inherently translate into the desired outcome. For example, while the implementation of the universal surgical checklist is globally accepted as the "gold standard" in operative patient safety [16], cases still occur where an entire operating room team "agrees" on an incorrect answer or team members fail to actively participate in the process. Such scenarios can easily become associated with retained surgical items or wrong-site surgeries [15, 17]. Consequently, lack of an appropriate championship, combined with a lack of appropriate team focus, can still produce disastrous consequences despite the most well-designed safety systems being in place. Finally, important lessons have been learned during the current coronavirus disease 2019 (COVID-19) pandemic [18, 19]. These lessons further inform our overall understanding of patient safety dynamics under the conditions of extreme healthcare system stress and acute resource limitations.

6. Synthesis and conclusion

In this book, we will explore new developments and evolving trends within the highly complex environment of patient safety, with a strong emphasis on the interrelationship between healthcare safety and quality of care. In addition to presenting various descriptive aspects of patient safety, the chapters enclosed herein also provide a perspective on how to approach different opportunities for improvement at the institutional level. The goal here is to strengthen existing patient safety systems and to facilitate the implementation of specific solutions while addressing major opportunities and concerns. Our key message is, and will continue to be, centered around the importance of teamwork, excellent communication, honest disclosure, and a non-punitive approach to systemic remedies. Only through well-coordinated educational and skill-building efforts, beginning with the earliest stages of medical education, then proceeding through graduate medical training, and finally continuing throughout one's healthcare career, can we build effective systems that will sustainably deliver high quality and the safest possible patient care.

Author details

James P. Orlando[1,2], Michael S. Firstenberg[3] and Stanislaw P. Stawicki[4*]

1 Department of Graduate Medical Education, St. Lukes University Health Network, USA

2 Graduate School of Education, University of Pennsylvania, USA

3 Department of Cardiothoracic and Vascular Surgery, Ascension St. Elizabeth Medical Center, Appleton, Wisconsin, USA

4 Department of Research and Innovation, St. Luke's University Health Network, Bethlehem, Pennsylvania, USA

*Address all correspondence to: stawicki.ace@gmail.com

References

[1] Laffel G, Blumenthal D. The case for using industrial quality management science in health care organizations. JAMA. 1989;**262**(20):2869-2873

[2] Stawicki S. Fundamentals of Patient Safety in Medicine and Surgery. Gurugram, Haryana, India: Wolters kluwer India Pvt Ltd.; 2015

[3] Stawicki SP et al. Introductory chapter: Patient safety is the cornerstone of modern healthcare delivery systems. Vignettes in Patient Safety. 2019;**4**:1-11

[4] Portner M et al. Learning from others: Examples from air transportation and industrial realms. In: Stawicki S et al., editors. Fundamentals of Patient Safety in Medicine and Surgery. New Delhi: Wolters Kluwer Health (India) Pvt Ltd; 2014

[5] Donabedian A. An Introduction to Quality Assurance in Health Care. Oxford, United Kingdom: Oxford University Press; 2002

[6] Ogrinc GS. Fundamentals of Health Care Improvement: A Guide to Improving Your Patient's Care. Oak Brook, IL, USA: Joint Commission Resources; 2012. Available from: https://www.jcrinc.com/about-us/

[7] Saeed M et al. Fact versus conjecture: Exploring levels of evidence in the context of patient safety and care quality. In: Vignettes in Patient Safety. Vol. 3. London, UK: IntechOpen; 2018

[8] Chen C, Petterson S, Phillips RL, Mullan F, Bazemore A, O'Donnell MS. Towards graduate medical education (GME) accountability: Measuring the outcomes of GME institutions. Academic Medicine: Journal of the Association of American Medical Colleges. 2013;**88**(9):1267. Available from: https://www.ncbi.nlm.nih.gov/pmc/articles/PMC3761381

[9] Asch DA et al. Evaluating obstetrical residency programs using patient outcomes. JAMA. 2009;**302**(12):1277-1283

[10] Hartz AJ, Kuhn EM, Pulido J. Prestige of training programs and experience of bypass surgeons as factors in adjusted patient mortality rates. Medical Care. 1999:93-103. Available from: https://www.jstor.org/stable/3767212

[11] Dartmouth_Atlas_Project. The Dartmouth Atlas of Health Care. 2021. Available from: https://www.dartmouthatlas.org/

[12] Carroll J, Rudolph J. Design of high reliability organizations in health care. BMJ Quality & Safety. 2006;**15** (suppl. 1):i4-i9

[13] Buist M. Adverse Events in Hospitals: "Swiss Cheese" Versus the "Hierarchal Referral Model of Care and Clinical Futile Cycles". In: Stawicki SP, Firstenberg MS, editors. Vignettes in Patient Safety. Vol. 3 [Internet]. London: IntechOpen; 2018. DOI: 10.5772/intechopen.75380. Available from: https://www.intechopen.com/chapters/60108 [cited 2022 Mar 07]

[14] Tolentino JC et al. Introductory chapter: Developing patient safety champions. In: Vignettes in Patient Safety. Vol. 2. London, UK: IntechOpen; 2018

[15] Lin A et al. Wrong-site procedures: Preventable never events that continue to happen. Vignettes in Patient Safety. 2018;**2**:2113

[16] Smith E et al. Surgical safety checklist: Productive, nondisruptive, and the "right thing to do". Journal of Postgraduate Medicine. 2015;**61**(3):214

[17] Stawicki SP et al. Natural history of retained surgical items supports the need

for team training, early recognition, and prompt retrieval. The American Journal of Surgery. 2014;**208**(1):65-72

[18] Papadimos TJ et al. COVID-19 blind spots: A consensus statement on the importance of competent political leadership and the need for public health cognizance. Journal of Global Infectious Diseases. 2020;**12**(4):167

[19] Stawicki SP et al. The 2019-2020 novel coronavirus (severe acute respiratory syndrome coronavirus 2) pandemic: A joint american college of academic international medicine-world academic council of emergency medicine multidisciplinary COVID-19 working group consensus paper. Journal of Global Infectious Diseases. 2020;**12**(2):47

Chapter 2

Patient Safety: Preventing Patient Harm and Building Capacity for Patient Safety

Gregory Domer, Thomas M. Gallagher, Shekiba Shahabzada, Juliana Sotherland, Elisabeth N. Paul, Kushee-Nidhi Kumar, Bryan Wilson, Shilpa Salpekar and Parampreet Kaur

Abstract

Patient safety is a global public health concern. It is a health care discipline with ever evolving advancement and complexity resulting in consequential rise in patient harm. Since the pandemic, patient safety has been threatened even more by laying bare the inadequacies of health systems. Many unsafe care practices, risks, and errors contribute to patient harm and overall economic burden. These include medical, diagnostic, and radiation errors, healthcare associated infections, unsafe surgical procedures and transfusion practices, sepsis, venous thromboembolism, and falls. Although patient safety has become an integral part of the healthcare delivery model and resources have been dedicated towards it, much still needs to be achieved. An attitude of inclusivity for all care teams and anyone in contact with the patient, including the patients themselves, would enhance patient safety. Incorporating this attitude from educational infancy will allow for better identification of medical errors and inculcate critical analysis of process improvement. Implementing the 'Just Culture' by health care organizations can build the infrastructure to eliminate avoidable harm. To reduce avoidable harm and improve safety, a constant flow of information and knowledge should be available to mitigate the risks. Lastly, proper communication and effective leadership can play an imperative role to engage stakeholders and reduce harm.

Keywords: Patient safety, medical errors, diagnostic errors, and radiation errors, healthcare associated infections, COVID-19 pandemic, unsafe surgical procedures, unsafe transfusion practices, sepsis, venous thromboembolism, falls, patient safety education

1. Introduction

"First, do no harm"- The Hippocratic Oath. Patient safety is pivotal to high-quality health care. The World Health Organization (WHO) defines patient safety as "a framework of organized activities that creates cultures, processes, procedures,

behaviors, technologies and environments in health care that consistently and sustainably lower risks, reduce the occurrence of avoidable harm, make error less likely and reduce its impact when it does occur" [1]. Ideally, the goal of all healthcare is zero preventable harm to patients, however, we are far from this target. Medical error is a global and system wide phenomenon which is present in all aspects of medicine and resources must be implemented at every level to recognize and limit its occurrence to improve patients' wellbeing. In this chapter, we will discuss topics that pose risks to patients in healthcare and ways systems and individuals can help mitigate them.

2. Reasons of patient harm

"To err is human"- Alexander Pope. Preventable medical errors can be attributed to several factors, including actions by healthcare professionals, systematic failures, or a combination of factors on multiple levels of care [2]. Although medical error is recognized as a leading cause of mortality worldwide, lack of reliable data at the organizational, national or international level, challenges in redesigning and implementing new healthcare systems, and difficulty engaging medical professionals in patient safety improvement activities contribute to continued lack of progress [3].

Certain healthcare settings and situations are also prone to higher levels of hazards and chances of error. For example, intensive care unit (ICU) patients' care is complex with multiple disciplines involved performing numerous activities and procedures that increase the potential risk of error [3]. A recent study reports that drug management (25%, 95% confidence interval 16% to 34%, I^2=98%) and other therapeutic management incidents (24%, 21% to 30%, I^2=98%), surgical procedures (23%, 9% to 38%, I^2=98%) and healthcare infections (16%, 11% to 22%, I^2=98%) are the leading causes of preventable patient harm [2, 4, 5]. Lastly, fear around reporting medical errors manifests strongly within the healthcare culture in numerous places around the world, and contributes to stunting advancement towards error prevention and patient safety [5].

3. The burdens of harm

Though patient safety is an essential principle of health care, yet many medical practices and risks related with healthcare are major challenges for patient safety. In high-income countries, one in 10 patients experiences an adverse event during their hospital stay [4]. In the United States, medical error is the third leading cause of death after cancer and heart disease, resulting in 250,000 deaths annually, and in the United Kingdom, a patient is reported to be harmed every 35 seconds [5, 6]. Low and middle-income countries fare far worse as one in four patients is estimated to be harmed, which results in 2.6 million yearly deaths [4].

Additionally, the cost of medical errors associated with poor care is an enormous economic burden. Unsafe practices which result in death or permanent disability have cost some countries between US $6 billion and US $29 billion per year [5]. Furthermore, the psychological cost to the patient and families associated with a loved one's death or disability, and loss of trust in the healthcare system are immeasurable [5]. Studies report that annual global economic growth could be boosted by over 0.7% if harmful medical practices are eliminated [4].

The joint commission gathers new evidence on emerging patient safety issues to inform goals for every year. Below are the brief descriptions of common safety issues, its burden, and the steps that can be taken to improve each.

3.1 Medical errors

Medical errors are events that occur during medical care which can lead to adverse consequences to patients. It is the third leading cause of death in the United States behind heart disease and cancer; about 250,000 deaths can be attributed to medical errors, including medication errors [7, 8]. They can be related to events when a wrong action was taken (error of commission) or when an action was not taken (error of omission). Additionally, medical errors can have consequences to health care professionals and institutions due to negative financial outcomes [9]. Healthcare providers can experience negative psychological responses with fear of punishment, and therefore be hesitant to report errors. It has been suggested that acknowledging healthcare providers are fallible and promoting a culture that focuses on mental health can lead to improved care for patients [10].

Several aspects of medical care can lead to medical error, including misdiagnosis, procedures, medication and/or dosage, patient identification and billing. It is important to recognize why they occur, foster a culture that encourages quality improvement, and cautions against an environment of blame and punishment [11]. There is often multiple causes of medical error: insufficient training, responsibilities performed by inappropriate staff, rare diseases, complexity of illness, unsatisfactory testing, time restraints, patient's age, and newer procedures, amongst others [7]. It is important for all members of the healthcare delivery team to be involved in all aspects of patient safety and improvement.

3.2 Diagnostic errors

Diagnostic errors have been estimated to be associated with up to 40,000 to 80,000 deaths or injuries per year. These include situations when a diagnosis was an unintentional delay, incorrect, or overlooked, and can occur in all specialties over a wide range of diagnoses. Preventing errors in diagnosis is a multifaceted approach, ranging from ensuring awareness of conditions that are often misdiagnosed, acknowledging first impression bias, discussion with appropriate specialists, and clear communication and documentation. This includes a complete differential diagnosis, appropriate handoffs, if applicable, and knowing which patients are at higher risks of diagnostic error, such as those with multiple medical conditions, patients with language and socioeconomic barriers, and patients with poor follow-up and compliance. Interventions to reduce diagnostic errors should not only be at the individual level, but should ideally be focused at the systems based level. System related errors include technical and equipment problems, organizational failures, "no-fault" errors like unusual presentation or conditions, and patient-related issues, such as compliance and misrepresenting symptom concerns [12–14].

The COVID-19 pandemic brings to light the importance of medical errors, including diagnostic errors as it relates to learning a new disease entity, as well as compromised physical and psychological aspects of healthcare providers that can affect clinical reasoning [15]. Additionally, system-based factors, such as staffing, capacity of the healthcare facility, and new care delivery systems, could be prone to delayed diagnosis due to postponement in patients coming to seek evaluation of symptoms or preventive screenings. It has been suggested that strategies to mitigate diagnostic error during these challenging times can be helpful: decision support tools, electronic health record, triage protocol, optimized use of telemedicine and follow-up, encouraging patients to seek care, education on safety protocols, a strong healthcare leadership team, open door for concerns without fear of judgement, continued support for education of trainees, and opportunities for discussion among colleagues for challenging cases and situations [16].

3.3 Sepsis

Sepsis is a syndrome characterized by life-threatening organ dysfunction in response to an infection. It is frequently not diagnosed early enough to save a patient's life. Because these infections are often resistant to antibiotics, patients are at high risk for complications and death and have higher health care costs [17]. **Sepsis** affects an estimated 31 million people worldwide and causes over 5 million deaths per year [18]. Even though there is a sepsis campaign guideline, the mortality from sepsis worldwide is still high at 34–46% [19]. The incidence of severe sepsis increases by approximately 13% each year in the United States, and it is a leading cause of morbidity and mortality worldwide [20]. Sepsis accounted for more than $20 billion or 5.2% of total hospital costs in year of 2011 alone in the United States [21].

In October 2015, the Centers for Medicare and Medicaid Services (CMS) began requiring U.S. hospitals to report compliance rates with the sepsis CMS core measure SEP-1 (Severe Sepsis and Septic Shock Management Bundle). It puts out guidelines for frontline hospital clinicians fighting sepsis. SEP-1 focuses on timely sepsis recognition and early intervention with lifesaving therapies [22]. Preliminary data from CMS indicate that the majority of SEP-1 cases nationally fail the measure and cases that fail have higher mortality rates than cases that pass [23]. E*ach hour of delay before a septic patient is treated is associated with a 4% increased risk of mortality*. In another multicenter retrospective cohort study, crude mortality rates were higher in sepsis cases that failed versus passed SEP-1 [24]. Early recognition and treatment of sepsis is associated with decreased mortality and improved patient outcomes.

3.4 Radiation errors

Radiation therapy, consisting of targeting malignant cells with ionized radiation, is an increasingly important cancer therapy with approximately 50% of all cancer patients receiving radiation during their illness [25]. Toxicities and adverse side effects of this therapy are related to the dose of radiation given and therefore dose calculation and regulation is of concern with regards to patient safety.

Radiation therapy safety and regulation has been under scrutiny and overhaul following a New York Times article from 2010 describing several patient stories with devastating outcomes [26, 27]. Many of the errors described are related to patients receiving several times the intended dose of radiation or miscalculations of the field resulting in areas of the body receiving radiation which were not intended or planned. Unfortunately, these errors are caused by flaws in an exceedingly complicated series of calculations and considerations depending heavily on computers systems and software. In fact, data shows that in radiation oncology, 30% of errors occur in the planning phase of therapy and 29% of errors are discovered in the treatment step of therapy [27]. This may suggest that the planning phase needs a more robust universally standardized control system and many studies have attempted to elucidate areas of improvement regarding geometric discrepancies resulting in errors [28–30].

As medicine becomes increasingly more complex, so does error analysis. In the field of radiation oncology, the multidisciplinary team adds to this complexity. The specific skill sets that are required to plan and execute a radiation treatment cannot be expected of one provider and so several health care providers are needed to successfully implement a complex therapy, including a highly specialized physician, medical physicist, and radiation therapist/dosimetrist. This is no doubt overall beneficial in the big picture for patient outcomes, however, advanced software and multiple highly specialized providers means that the way providers consider their options when an image or patient is in front of them requires far more critical thinking than what may have been expected from an average physician 30 years ago. Each provider must critically look at the information in front of them and understand and accept that there are parts of the treatment plan and the method in which they were derived that they do not fully comprehend. This requires all the members of the treatment team to trust the computer systems and software, as well as other providers, which are all integral in planning of radiation therapy. At the same time, all involved must realize the limitations of technology and consider human error on the part of their colleagues. This makes error analysis in the field of radiation oncology intricate, and one might argue that a key consideration in the future may be cognitive biases among providers and need for structured training to minimize them [27].

3.5 Unsafe surgical practices

Every year, millions of people undergo surgical treatment for various ailments and disease processes. Surgical interventions account for an estimated 13% of the world's total disability-adjusted life years (DALYs). These procedures are intended to improve and save lives; however, unsafe surgical care can cause substantial harm. A modeling study, published in Lancet in 2008, estimated that 234 million operations are carried out every year across the world [31]. This translates to one operation for every 25 people, which is more than the number of children born worldwide each year. Current estimates of morbidity and mortality following surgery indicate that over 7 million people (about twice the population of Oklahoma) worldwide will suffer complications following surgery. One million of these people will die as a result. This correlates to an overall mortality rate of 0.5-5%. Complications in inpatient operations occur in up to 25% of our patients, which accounts for nearly half of all adverse events in hospitalized patients [31]. Regrettably, it is estimated that in at least half of the cases, in which surgery led to harm, were considered preventable. Several surgical societies and hospital administrations have put forth recommendations, and in many cases requirements, to help ensure our patients have a safe journey through our operating rooms.

On a global scale, the World Health Organization (WHO) is the leading authority on patient safety and has undertaken essential global and regional initiatives to address surgical safety. WHO established the Second Global Patient Safety Challenge, "Safe Surgery Saves Lives," in 2007. This program proposed to improve the safety of surgical care around the world by defining a core set of safety standards which led to the Surgical Safety Checklist, a 19-item tool created by WHO in association with the Harvard School of Public Health. This safety checklist aims to decrease errors and adverse events by increasing communication and teamwork in surgery [32]. Improving teamwork and communication is one of the main goals of using a checklist. The checklist is a simple tool designed to improve the safety of surgical procedures by bringing together the whole operating team (surgeons, anesthesia providers and nurses) to perform key safety checks during vital phases of perioperative care: prior to the induction of anesthesia, prior to skin incision, and before the team leaves the operating room. Between October 2007 and September 2008, the effect of the Checklist was studied in eight hospitals in eight cities (Toronto, Canada; New Delhi, India; Amman, Jordan; Auckland, New Zealand; Manila, The Philippines; Ifakara, Tanzania; London, UK; and Seattle, USA) representing a wide variety of health-care settings, economic circumstances and diverse patient populations and demonstrated dramatic improvements in both processes and outcomes. The study showed use of the WHO Surgery Checklist, reduced the rate of deaths and surgical complications by more than one-third across all eight pilot hospitals. The rate of major inpatient complications dropped from 11% to 7%, and the inpatient death rate following major operations fell from 1.5% to 0.8% [33].

Many hospitals are already performing most of the items on the list but not reviewing them as a team. Good data has now proven that implementation of the 19-item checklist results in a significant reduction in both morbidity and mortality [33]. The WHO continues to develop patient safety action plans with an action-oriented framework to facilitate the implementation of strategic patient safety interventions at all levels of health systems. Because complications will strike, we must strive for perfection, by adhering to proven protocols, meticulously preparing, conducting, and caring for our surgical patients.

3.6 Blood transfusion safety

Each day, life-saving blood transfusions are needed in hospitals and emergency treatment facilities across the United States. There are more than 13.2 million blood donors in the U.S., resulting in a total of 17.2 million transfused blood product units per year. Worldwide, approximately 118.5 million blood donations are collected [34]. How do we ensure safety with this staggering number? In the U.S., the federal agencies responsible for keeping our blood safe are the Centers for Disease Control (CDC), protecting health through investigations and surveillance [35]. The U.S. Food and Drug Administration (FDA) ensures safety of blood donations by protecting the health of donors. The National Institutes of Health (NIH) performs research on blood transfusion basic science, epidemiology, and clinical practices. Safety is also the responsibility of the blood centers and hospitals that collect and transfuse millions of units of blood each year. On the donor end, each donor is screened for risk of transmissible disease by questionnaire, which asks standard health questions to determine eligibility to donate. Additionally, each unit of donated blood in the U.S. is routinely screened for various infectious disease pathogens, using FDA approved assays [35]. The blood is then tested for blood type (ABO group) and Rh type (positive or negative). Prior to transfusion, the donor and blood unit are also tested for certain proteins (antibodies) that may cause adverse reactions in a person receiving a blood transfusion.

Presently, the most significant risk for a transfusion complication occurs due to noninfectious hazards from deficient processes [36]. The goal of providing safe transfusion therapy depends on a complex process that requires integration and coordination among multiple hospital services, including laboratory medicine, nursing, anesthesia, surgery, clerical support, and transportation. Most healthcare institutions in the United States have formed a multidisciplinary hospital-based transfusion committee to review blood transfusion practices and adverse outcomes. The Center for Medicare/Medicaid Services (CMS) requires such a process to receive payment for transfusion services. However, CMS does not require a specific committee be assigned to oversee the review process. This process must include a program of quality assessment and performance improvement, which is ongoing, hospital-wide, data-driven, reflects the complexity of the hospital's organization and services, and involves all hospital departments and services (including those contracted) [37]. If a hospital elects not to receive payments from Medicare, it must still comply with applicable sections of the Code of Federal Regulations pertaining to transfusion services.

3.7 Venous thromboembolism

Venous thromboembolism (VTE) is a frequent complication of hospitalized patients and a leading cause of preventable hospital death and increased hospital length of stay in the United States and worldwide. Hospital-acquired VTE is defined as VTE occurring during or within 3 months after hospitalization and accounts for >50% of the population burden of VTE in the United States. Although, the precise number of people affected by VTE is unknown, it is estimated as many as 900,000 people are affected (1 to 2 per 1,000) each year in the United States, resulting in an estimated loss of 60,000-100,000 American lives. As one might expect, there is an exponential increase with age from 1 per 10,000 in young adults to 1 per 100 in the elderly. Data from two large U.S. studies place the estimated absolute risk of VTE after age 45 to be 8.1% overall, 10.9% in obese patients, 11.5% in blacks, 17.1% in those with factor V Leiden mutation, and 18.2% among blacks with sickle cell trait [38]. Of these patients, two-thirds will present with Deep Vein Thrombosis (DVT) only and the remaining presenting with Pulmonary Embolism (PE) as the first manifestation and primary cause of VTE related mortality.

Early data regarding COVID-19 patients developing VTE suggests substantial risk. Reports have ranged from 1.1% in non–intensive care unit (ICU) hospital wards to 69% in ICU patients. More data is necessary regarding the relationship between COVID-19 and increased risk of VTE. Currently, many of reports are from small sample sizes and retrospective in design. However, it seems prudent that all patients admitted to a hospital unit receive pharmacologic prophylaxis. The question of whether to administer full therapeutic dose versus prophylactic dose anticoagulant in critically ill patients is controversial and is actively being studied [39].

Venous thromboembolism remains one of the most preventable causes of hospitalized patients. Risk stratification and prophylactic measures have proven to be safe, cost effective, and most importantly, save lives. The data regarding VTE morbidity and mortality is not new yet, despite decades of solid evidence from multiple randomized clinical trials, thromboprophylaxis remains either underused or misused. The key is for health care providers to adhere to proven protocols and policies. Multiple policy statements have been published focusing efforts to eliminate unnecessary human death and suffering. Five major areas of policy guidance have put forth by the American Heart Association that they believe will lead to improved implementation, tracking and prevention of VTE events. They include assessment and reporting the level of VTE risk in all hospitalized patients, integrating preventable VTE as a benchmark for hospital comparison and pay-for-performance programs, supporting appropriation to improve public awareness of VTE, tracking VTE nationwide with the use of standardized definition and developing a centralized data steward for data tracking on VTE risk assessment, prophylaxis, and rates [40].

Diagnosis and defining exactly who should be screened remains challenging because the clinical features are often non-specific, and testing can be falsely negative or positive. Therefore, risk stratification scoring systems have been proposed and used widely. The Wells DVT and Wells PE scoring systems, as well as the Geneva PE score, have been adopted by many major medical centers in the U.S. and around the world. These scoring systems have been used in conjunction with objective diagnostic imaging, providing a high degree of accuracy in making the diagnosis of VTE. Some of these diagnostic testing modalities includes compression ultrasonography, computed tomography angiography, ventilation-perfusion scintigraphy or single-photon emission tomography, magnetic resonance angiography and echocardiography.

Another method of making healthcare administrator's and medical practitioners take notice is by making them financially aware of the devasting avoidable cost to our healthcare industry. When factoring in the VTE-related morbidity of VTE, including post-phlebitic syndrome occurring in 30-50% of patients with proximal DVT, and chronic thromboembolic pulmonary hypertension occurring in 4% of patients within 2 years of PE survival, the estimated annual cost of preventable hospital acquired VTE is $7-10 billion per year [41]. Regardless of the method, it is our duty as healthcare providers to take on the challenge by educating our healthcare colleagues and soliciting the support of our administrators in establishing hospital wide protocols to prevent this devastating, albeit preventable, disease process.

3.8 Healthcare associated infections

Health-care associated infections (HCAIs) are infections acquired by patients 48 hours or more to within 30 days after receiving care from various health care settings, which include acute-care facility, long-term facility, family medicine clinics, ambulatory care and home care [42]. HCAIs are the most common complications of hospital care and one of the top 10 causes of mortality worldwide [42]. Numerous factors heighten the risk for developing HCAIs, such as increased age, immunosuppression, multiple underlying comorbidities, increased length of hospital stay, admission to the intensive care unit (ICU), mechanical ventilatory support, recent invasive procedures, indwelling devices, frequent visits to healthcare facilities, and infection-control practices at the healthcare facility [43]. Patients' risk of developing antimicrobial resistance increases highly if they received intravenous antibiotics within 90 days of administration [43]. Even though $28-45 billion is spent annually in the United States, 90,000 deaths still occur due to HCAIs [42]. The World Health Organization (WHO) reports that 7 out of 100 hospital patients in high income countries and 10 out of 100 hospital patients in low-to-middle income countries will acquire HCAIs at any given time [44]. These statistics continue to highlight a major concern to patient safety worldwide.

Surgical site infections (SSIs), also known as wound infections, central line-associated bloodstream infections (CLABSIs), catheter-associated urinary tract infections (CAUTIs), ventilator-associated pneumonia (VAP), hospital-acquired pneumonia (HAP) and *Clostridioides difficile* infections are the most common types of HCAIs [42, 43]. Most are caused by about 22 microorganisms, including Gram-positive bacteria, Gram-negative bacteria, fungal and viral species [42, 43, 45–48]. Formation of mono-or-poly-microorganism biofilms on indwelling devices or surgical wounds is also a major cause of resistant HCAIs [47].

The most important practice to prevent and control HCAIs is effective hand hygiene [42, 49]. The World Health Organization (WHO) advocates education and training for all healthcare workers to encourage washing hands for at least 30 seconds before and after touching a patient or their environment, after body fluid exposure, and before and after aseptic procedures using soap and water or alcohol-based sanitizers [42, 49]. Widespread and consistent hand hygiene practices can decrease infection rates by 50% [49].

Personal protective equipment (PPE), for example, face masks, gloves, gowns, protective eyewear, and face shields, reduce transmission of microorganisms and body fluids between healthcare workers and patients [42]. Organisms transmitted through aerosols, such as influenza virus, *Hemophilus influenzae*, and *Neisseria meningitidis*, are dispersed easily through droplets from one person to another in closed settings [42]. The most recent notable example of a highly transmissible respiratory virus is SARS-CoV-2, a type of coronavirus that caused COVID-19, emerged in 2019 and was responsible for a global pandemic which continued for more than a year and lead to millions of deaths worldwide. Basic handwashing for 30 seconds or using an alcohol-based hand sanitizer, use of face masks covering the nose and mouth, social distancing of at least 6 feet amongst people and proper ventilation of indoor spaces are largely attributed to the control of the pandemic [50]. Another very important factor was mRNA COVID-19 vaccinations against the virus among frontline healthcare workers and the greater community, starting with the most vulnerable, such as nursing home residents, people older than 75, essential workers, and patients with underlying health conditions, for example, cancer, diabetes type 1 and 2, and chronic lung diseases [50–52].

Cleanliness of equipment used by healthcare workers is also important to patient safety. A study found medical residents' coat sleeves (50%), stethoscopes (36.3%), and pagers (36.3%) carried methicillin sensitive *Staphylococcus aureus* (MSSA) and serve as potential sources of nosocomial transmission of pathogens to vulnerable patients [53]. High-touch surfaces by patients and staff in hospitals should be decontaminated with appropriate products as regularly as possible, especially bedrails, over-bed tables, call buttons, and reusable patient-care equipment [47]. Continued staff education and training about personal and environmental hygiene cannot be overstated and significantly contribute towards patient safety.

3.9 Falls

The estimated number of inpatient falls in United States is between 700,000 to 1,000,000, with reported fall rates ranging from 1.3 to 8.9 per 1000 bed-days [54, 55]. In general, fall related injuries are the most common cause of accidental death among hospital patients over 65, resulting in 41 fall-related deaths per 100,000 people per year [54].

Per the World Health Organization, falls are defined as "inadvertently coming to rest on the ground, floor, or other lower level, excluding intentional change in position" and in the inpatient setting, they include slips, trips, faints, collapses and any patient found on the floor unwitnessed [56]. As of 2008, Centers for Medicare & Medicaid Services (CMS) does not reimburse hospital for certain types of traumatic injuries while patients are in the hospital, many of which occur after a fall [57].

Preventing falls in the hospital setting can be challenging. Hospital staff needs to treat patient for their acute condition, keep them safe and help patients maintain and recover physically and mentally. When an adverse event like a fall happens, it may result in high-impact outcomes for a patient, such as decline in function, increased length of hospital stays, and increased cost of health care services. Damage resulting from a fall can affect as many as 50% of patients, and about 44% of falls can result in serious injuries and even death [56]. About 1-3% of falls in hospitals results in fractures [58]. Even without injury, harm to patients, caregivers and hospital staff can manifest as psychological distress, including anxiety and depression, reduced physical activity, fear of future falls, prolonged hospital stay, increased use of restrains and sedating drugs, complaints, litigations, guilt, and dissatisfaction [55, 59]. Fall prevention often consists of managing patients' underlying fall risk factors. Such risk factors include age, limited mobility, visual impairment, use of some classes of medications (especially psychotropics), medication side effects, change in medications, delirium, change in environment, frequent toilet needs, urinary incontinence, orthostatic hypotension, fall history, and fear of falling. In addition to the elderly, patients with recent diagnoses of stroke or cancer, and patients hospitalized in neurology and rehabilitation units are at increased risk of falls [60]. There are several fall-risk tools to help stratify patients at risk, but many of them are not validated due to their lack of sensitivity and specificity for clinical use. Three of these have been validated in multiple studies across the populations. These are the St Thomas's Risk Assessment Tool in Falling Elderly Inpatients (STRATIFY), the Morse Fall Scale (MFS), and the Hendrich Fall Risk Model (HFRM). Based on the risk stratification, there is usually a multimodal intervention for inpatient fall prevention, and it can include patient education, bedside risk sign, staff education, alert wristband, footwear, toileting schedules, environmental modifications, movement alarms, bedrail review, hip protection, exercise, restrains, and a review after a fall to identify causes. High quality evidence shows that multi-component intervention can reduce the risk of inpatient falls by up to 30% [61].

4. Key terms in patient safety

A common taxonomy is needed to standardize and track events to measure particularly when healthcare workers are working between and within different professional backgrounds. The core terms that are essential to know and understand are described below.

Sentinel Event: A patient safety event (not primarily related to the natural course of the patient's illness or underlying condition) that reaches a patient and results in any of the following: death; permanent harm; severe temporary harm. The Sentinel Event Policy explains how The Joint Commission partners with hospitals that have experienced a serious patient safety event to protect the patient, improve systems, and prevent further harm.

Safety Patient Events: An event incident, or condition that could have resulted or did result in harm to a patient. A patient safety event can be, but is not necessarily, the result of a defective system or process design, a system breakdown, equipment failure, or human error.

Adverse Events: Any untoward or unfavorable medical occurrence in a human subject, including any abnormal sign (for example, abnormal physical exam or laboratory finding), symptom or disease temporally associated with the subject's participation in the research.

Near Miss, Near Hit, Close Call or Nearly a Collision: An unplanned event that has the potential to cause, but does not actually result in human injury, environmental or equipment damage, or an interruption to normal operation.

Near misses also may be referred to as close calls, near accidents, accident precursors, injury-free events and, in the case of moving objects, near collisions.

A near miss is often an error, with harm prevented by other considerations and circumstances.

The phrase "near miss" should not be confused with the phrase “nearly a miss” which would imply a collision.

A No-Harm Event: A patient safety event that reaches the patient but does not cause harm. A close call (or “near miss” or “good catch”) is a patient safety event that did not reach the patient. Unsafe conditions are hazards that have the potential to cause injury or death to an employee. Some of these hazards include erroneous safety procedures, malfunctioning equipment or tools, or failure to utilize necessary safety equipment, such as goggles and masks.

5. Building capacity to change and proactive approach to preventing harm

A coordinated and practical strategy in which systemwide safety processes are applied across entire healthcare fields through collaboration among diverse stakeholders has been proven to provide the best outcomes. Risks are to be expected as healthcare is and will continue to be an ever evolving. Preventing harm and improving systems will not happen in a vacuum. It takes effort from frontline personnel, educators, trainers, and organizational leaders to create a systemwide approach. In the following section, we will discuss how we can prevent harm with our proactive attitude and build a capacity to improve patient safety when we try to conquer risks and errors spanning the myriad layers of healthcare.

DOI: http://dx.doi.org/10.5772/intechopen.100559

5.1 Education and training

The crucial step towards lowering errors and harms to the patients is educating healthcare professionals about patient safety. Since there is involvement of many individuals at different layers of the system in the delivery of health services, education and training also needs to be multidisciplinary and multi -professional. Education cannot be based on a linear or hierarchical educational model as medicine is often approached. Multimodal approach should be implemented at each level of health professional education.

Association of American Medical Colleges (AAMC) addressed Competency Based Education (CBE) in 2019 with suggestions for improvement for patient safety education. It acknowledges the importance of developing curricula based on competency at each level of learning- undergraduate, graduate, and continued education [62]. The same look but from a distinct perspective - as one accrues knowledge, they begin to see more clearly the finer aspects of how to prevent harm. Multiple avenues exist for formal coursework in patient safety education. Continued Medical Education (CME) is available by multiple formats such as lectures, testing, reading materials. It is the most pervasive patient safety education model; not only does updating clinical knowledge leads to improved outcomes but direct patient safety courses enhance its implementation. Certification courses are available, as well. In recent years there has been as rise in Master's degrees in patient safety and healthcare quality.

Several ongoing activities for trainees and experts, either directly or indirectly, enable patient safety education. Accreditation Council for Graduate Medical Education (ACGME) has mandated Quality Improvement (QI) projects in residency. They require pattern recognition for process improvement, inadvertently propelling involved parties to become educated on areas of patient harm. ACGME has appropriately made QI a requirement in physician training [63]. More informally, training occurs in the break rooms or during lunch when knowledge is shared openly, and indirect learning occurs from other's experience. The table below provides list of some of the pros, cons, and growth opportunities for each educational setting (**Table 1**).

WHO has recognized the need for an international leader in patient safety education. In 2013, WHO published a Multi-professional Patient Safety Curriculum Guide for standardization of patient safety education, an update to its earlier Curriculum Guide for Medical Schools published in 2009 [64]. Additionally, during their 2021 assembly, the WHO adopted the first ever Global Patient Safety Action Plan 2021 – 2030, a global initiative to eliminate avoidable harm. Amongst other things, it will focus on involving patients and families for patient safety [44]. Smaller entities, such as Improvement for Healthcare Safety (IHI) or Patient Safety Network (PSNET), have perceived this necessity and invested in producing a concise platform for medical professionals as well [65, 66] attempting to innovate this field of learning.

Having recognized the need for such courses in medical educational infancy, the new trend has been to incorporate patient safety education across the globe [67]. By creating patient safety education early on, lifelong learners of patient safety can be made.

COVID-19 pandemic has provided fertile ground for medical errors as the medical system was stretched thin [68]. Much learning and teaching had internationally shifted to the virtual world. If this shift can be harnessed to standardize patient safety education as we continue to grapple with COVID as a reference, it may allow us to build a more robust patient safety instruction. Updating courses in medical school to incorporate patient safety is a new trend [69]. While each organization and individual will need to adapt proposed training, interactive learning curriculums improve student learning of difficult concepts such as patient safety and "just

Type	Description	Pros	Cons	Potential sources of improvement
M&M conference	Healthcare teams thoroughly analyze a case often using the Ishikawa Diagram to discuss errors with an audience to educate and identify improvement	1. Involves root cause analysis of errors involving multiple factors from system to individual 2. Nonjudgmental review of errors 3. Residents /Fellows are involved in M&M committees	1. Can devolve into blame-oriented discussion	1. Pursue effective implementation of learnings from a case
QI projects	Process improvement using the PDSA cycle	1. Improves critical thinking analysis for process improvement to prevent errors 2. Can be multidisciplinary 3. Mandated in residency 4. Addresses evolving nature of medicine 5. Improves vigilance for patient care	1. Administrative obstacles may delay improvement in processes thus potentially allowing for preventable patient harm 2. Disinterest in project after implementation may lead to loss of an opportunity for process improvement leading to continued errors	1. Publish/share positive AND negative findings within systems/ nationwide/ worldwide
Case analysis	Experts reviewers who are familiar to the system and individuals find issues leading to patient harm	1. If internal, usually experts reviewers are familiar to the system and individuals so can provided enhanced insight to prevent of future errors 2. Can lead to learner/expert specific improvements for typical and atypical cases	1. Reviewer specific identification of errors 2. Retrospective review can miss factors present at time of decision making 3. Can lead to blame oriented identification of errors	1. Apply case analysis at all levels of education and not just as a part of M&M
CME	Short formal sessions on specific topics on patient safety	1. Multimodal 2. Universal approach to complete provider requirements	1. Can be dated 2. Learners can lose interest usually if in non-interactive format/because it is mandatory	1. Create interactive sessions/ simulations to showcase patient safety

Type	Description	Pros	Cons	Potential sources of improvement
Courses	Longer formal training on specific topics on patient safety	1. Multimodal 2. Allows time for in depth dive into patient safety for greater understanding	1. Long time commitment required for completion 2. May be taught by non-clinical staff 3. Usually, didactic teaching	1. Mandate instructors to have ongoing patient contact so teaching can better tailor for real world timely application
Multidisciplinary rounds	Involve multiple patient team member-such as provider, nurse, pharmacist, residents, fellows, etc to oversee patient care and provide increased oversight to prevent patient harm	1. Dynamic discourse allows each to provide teaching from the perspective of their role for patient safety 2. A platform for patient safety and education innovation 3. Trainees directly or inadvertently can learn to keep patient safer by listening to diverse team members	1. Can be uninviting to innovative ideas/teaching depending on discussion leader	1. Prompt providers and even other clinical staff to discuss new advances in methods to prevent patient harm 2. Provide infrastructure for more multidisciplinary rounds
Books/Articles/ News	Dedicated books on/patient-oriented perspectiveopinions on patient safety	1. Fresh and new perspectives on errors 2. Can highlight changing nature of patient safety 3. Books can provide a well thought of, comprehensive view on patient safety	1. Biased understanding of patient errors as non-clinical or uninvolved persons may be writing 2. Lengthy reads not always suitable for patient facing staff	1. A less litigious society would provide a better platform for open discussion in literature

Table 1.
Avenues for patient safety education.

culture". With the correct attitude, continually renewed educational offerings, and standardization of basics globally, we can navigate the complex and evolving nature of medicine better.

5.2 Role of healthcare organization leaders in patient safety

Effective leadership is necessary to lead an organization down the path to establishing a culture of safety. Primarily, the leadership needs to be persistent and well-balanced. Stable organizational leadership allows organizations to grow and transform successfully. According to the American College of Healthcare Executives and the Lucian Leape Institute, there are 6 key domains that healthcare leaders need to focus on to create a long-lasting organizational culture of safety [70]:

1. Establishing a compelling vision for safety

2. Build trust, respect, and inclusion

3. Select, develop, and engage your Board

4. Prioritize safety in the selection and development of leaders

5. Lead and reward a just culture

6. Establish organizational behavior expectations

These domains do not exist by themselves and must always be looked at as a cohesive unit.

To successfully lead an organization on its path to a safer patient experience, the leader must set clear priorities and communicate a sharp vision. A shared vision is a fundamental part of highly effective organizations, and this endeavor is no different. Because so much of patient safety initiatives involves voluntary reporting by staff, the role of leadership building trust amongst their employees and selecting managers who prioritize safety cannot be understated. Many staff members view patient safety reports as "snitching" and do not understand the fundamental importance of identifying these sentinel events. Leaders and managers leading by example in reporting events concerning them and by ensuring the principles of "just culture" are on display is necessary to ensuring the organization becomes a champion for patient safety.

The pairing of high-quality education and transformative leadership based on the 6 domains are two-parts to a successful, patient-focused organization. Neither will be successful alone and without coordination of educational programming and leadership efforts, they will not be successful either. Leaders will need to work with organization educational designers to create engage, transformative educational material that will motivate staff to focus on patient safety as a core value of the organization [71].

5.3 A fair and just culture

"Just Culture" refers to a system of shared accountability in which organizations are accountable for the systems they have designed and for responding to the behaviors of their employees in a fair and just manner. Employees are accountable for the quality of their choices and for reporting errors and system vulnerabilities. While the organization has a duty and responsibility to employees and to patients, all employees are held responsible for the quality of their choices [72].

Promoting a just culture is to implement a nonpunitive response to error in improving patient outcome and safety. Just culture encourages employee to focus on compliance and corrective actions instead of fear of punitive actions. Creating a safe and transparent environment encourages reporting of mistakes and hazards and improves the care provided to patients. Lack of reported information decreases the organization ability to proactively address patient-safety issues and improves the existing work infrastructure.

For health care systems to be successful in achieving the above goals of patient safety they need to foster a just culture [72].

These examples address an aspect of just culture that goes beyond ensuring that employees feel free to report errors. Exceptionally reliable organizations and industries promote mindfulness in their workers.

Weick and Sutcliffe describe mindfulness in terms of 5 components [73]:

1. A constant concern about the possibility of failure

2. Deference to expertise regardless of rank or status

3. Ability to adapt when the unexpected occurs

4. Ability to concentrate on a task while having a sense of the big picture

5. Ability to alter and flatten the hierarchy to fit a specific situation

Mindfulness throughout an organization considers moves beyond events and occurrences. Everyone in the organization is continually learning, adjusting, and redesigning systems for safety and managing behavioral choices.

A fair and just culture improves patient safety by empowering employees to proactively monitor the workplace and participate in safety efforts in the work environment. Improving patient safety reduces risk by its focus on managing human behavior (or helping others to manage their own behavior) and redesigning systems. In a just culture, employees are not only accountable for their actions and choices, but they are also accountable to each other, which may help some overcome the inherent resistance to dealing with incompetency [72].

Secondary benefits of a just culture include the ability to develop a positive patient safety profile to respond to outside auditors, such as The Joint Commission. When implemented, a just culture fosters innovation and cross-departmental communication. An example is the opportunity to revitalize the morbidity and mortality conference to cross specialty lines and develop a patient-centered focus. In a just culture, both the organization and its people are held accountable while focusing on risk, systems design, human behavior, and patient safety [72].

The process of implementing the just culture is not one that happens overnight. However, a health care organization can build an infrastructure to embed this methodology by achieving it through education and allocation of resources to training the employee.

5.4 Patient engagement

"Engagement of patients and families resides at the core of the framework for safe, reliable, and effective care. In safe and reliable organizations, patients and families are as much members of the care team as clinicians and other health care staff" [74].

The joint commission mandated that healthcare organizations "encourage patient's active involvement in their own care as a patient safety strategy". Because of this action, hospitalized patients, as well as patients receiving care on outpatient basis, are routinely surveyed about their satisfaction with the care they received [75].

Studies in the in-patient setting have found that patients often report errors that were not detected through traditional mechanisms, such as chart review [75]. Unless patient involvement through surveys after service was considered, these errors would not have been detected. Therefore, patient engagement and involvement practices in the day-to-day functions of an organization is essential in ensuring a safe environment.

Some examples of safety targets in patient care that show patient outcome improvement and risk reduction through patient engagement in hospitals and outpatient settings include: improved anticoagulation management with reduction in risks of thromboembolic events and mortality, improved hypoglycemia management in diabetes, increased medication adherence, reduced medication administration errors, improved hospital readmissions rates, and reduced hospital acquired infections when patient education and engagement is optimized and encouraged [76].

With all the evidence demonstrating patient involvement and participation supporting positive outcome, the next step is for health care teams to partner with patients and caregivers to integrate effective patient engagement into clinical practice and health care systems.

The following elaborates on proposed methods to involve and engage patients in the care they receive from organizations to ensure patient satisfaction and safety outcomes [74]:

1. Patients should be included in decision making process. While it is the clinical team's responsibility to provide key facts and advise to patients, the patients and/or their representatives should be given opportunity to have input in decision-making process. It is easier to reach a common goal when all parties are informed and well educated on real expectations. This will minimize unnecessary steps and reduced risks and negative outcomes associated with those steps.

2. Healthcare teams and organizations should provide a safe environment for patients to express concerns, questions, and ideas openly and without judgment. The clinical team should avoid negative reactions to foster more comprehensive and accurate information exchange between patients and organizations/healthcare teams. As a result, patients will be more forthcoming about their incompliances and will provide more accurate information. This process will help providers utilize factual data to come up with a plan of care that reduces unintentional harm to patients.

5.5 Agency for healthcare research and quality (AHRQ)

The Agency for Healthcare Research and Quality (AHRQ) is one of twelve agencies within US Department of Health and Human services (HHS). It is a lead federal agency charged with improving the quality and safety of America's health system performance, offers practical and research-based tools with resources to support healthcare organizations, providers, hospital staff, patients and others that make care safer in healthcare settings. These organized tools and resources help staff in hospitals, emergency departments, long-term care facilities, and ambulatory settings to prevent avoidable complications of care. AHRQ contributes to forming a higher performing health system in three main ways: investing in research and evidence to improve safety and quality of healthcare, creating materials to teach and train healthcare professionals to catalyze the improvements in care, and generating measures and data used to track and evaluate progress of US healthcare [77].

AHRQ assists and provides various tools and resources by different settings, quality measures, reports and resources, engaging patients and families, education, and training, etc. Teams STEPPS, is one such teamwork system developed by AHRQ and Department of Defense (DoD) that offers a powerful solution to improving collaboration and communication among healthcare professionals [78]. There are many other quality improvement tools and information, including AHRQ Quality Indicators Hospital Toolkit, ambulatory clinical performance measures, and talking quality, to help staff build the knowledge and develop the skills that impact organizational culture and lead to sustained improvements in safety.

5.6 Effective use of data (collecting, analyzing, using to drive improvement)

Since quality improvement is a driving force and is a vital part at every level of service delivery in healthcare, collecting and analyzing data are therefore central to the function of quality improvement at all levels. Data not only allows us to accurately recognize problems, it also supports to prioritize quality improvement initiatives, and qualifies objective assessment of whether change and improvement have indeed occurred. Making changes to improve quality is complex business, thus solid evidence in the form of data is required to support decision-making rather than isolated occurrences, assumptions, emotions, or politics.

Role of data in quality improvement is helpful in all five phases of quality improvement: project definition phase (what is the problem?), diagnosis phase (what can we improve?), intervention phase (how can we achieve improvement?), impact measurement phase (have we achieved improvement?), and sustainability phase (have we sustained improvement?) [79].

With good data, we can access: current performance, identify performance gaps, identify problem steps, prioritize opportunities for improvements, establish clear objectives for improvement, prioritize most appropriate interventions, compare the benefits of alternative interventions and implementation strategies, assess impacts of interventions, demonstrate the success of improvement project to stakeholders, provide feedback to reinforce change, demonstrate benefits, identify problems in practice, and need for repeated intervention.

To get quality, unbiased data, one must use sound data collection techniques, appropriate tools, correct sampling techniques, ensure data validity, and confirm it is secured.

6. Conclusion

The dynamic nature of healthcare delivery where innovative technologies and approaches to care are incorporated constantly into the regular practice, new occasions for unsafe practices are continually created. An attitude of inclusivity for all care teams with necessary education, proper communication, just culture, and engaging leadership will lower errors and harms and improve patient safety. Besides these, proper collection and review of safety data can help serve as a catalyst for increased resources dedication to most needed facet of healthcare in that setup. Thus, if we integrate the science of safety into our daily healthcare practices, we are certain to lessen the magnitude and extent of harm and economic burden and improve patient safety.

Author details

Gregory Domer[1], Thomas M. Gallagher[2], Shekiba Shahabzada[3], Juliana Sotherland[4], Elisabeth N. Paul[5], Kushee-Nidhi Kumar[6], Bryan Wilson[7], Shilpa Salpekar[8] and Parampreet Kaur[1*]

1 St. Luke's University Health Network, Temple University, Bethlehem, USA

2 Department of Medicine, St. Luke's University Health Network, Lewis Katz School of Medicine at Temple University, Bethlehem, USA

3 Core Faculty, Department of Family Medicine Residency Anderson, St. Luke's University Health Network, Temple University, Bethlehem, USA

4 Department of Internal Medicine Residency Anderson, St. Luke's University Health Network, Temple University, Bethlehem, USA

5 Hospitalist Faculty, Department of Internal Medicine Residency Anderson, St. Luke's University Health Network, Temple University, Bethlehem, USA

6 Department of Research and Innovation, St. Luke's University Health Network, Temple University, Bethlehem, USA

7 Core Faculty, Department of Emergency Medicine Residency Anderson, St. Luke's University Health Network, Temple University, Bethlehem, USA

8 Resident PGY II Department of Internal Medicine Residency Anderson, St. Luke's University Health Network, Temple University, Bethlehem, USA

*Address all correspondence to: parampreet.kaur@sluhn.org

References

[1] WHO. What is patient safety?" Patient Safety. World Health Organization. 12 June 2021.

[2] Panagioti M, Khan K, Keers RN, Abuzour A, Phipps D, Kontopantelis E, et al. Prevalence, severity, and nature of preventable patient harm across medical care settings: systematic review and meta-analysis. BMJ. 2019;**366**:l4185

[3] Carayon P, Wood KE. Patient safety - the role of human factors and systems engineering. Studies in health technology and informatics. 2010;**153**: 23-46

[4] Donaldson S. Dhingra, N, Gupta, N. et al. Towards Eliminating avoidable harm in health care World Health Organization.

[5] World Health O. Patient safety: making health care safer. Geneva: World Health Organization; 2017 2017. Contract No.: WHO/HIS/SDS/2017.11.

[6] Bartman T, Bertoni CB, Merandi J, Brady M, Bode RS. Patient Safety: What Is Working and Why? Current Treatment Options in Pediatrics. 2019;**5**(2):131-144

[7] Carver N GV, Hipskind JE. Medical Error. [Updated 2021 Jul 9]. StatPearls [Internet]: Treasure Island (FL): StatPearls Publishing; 2021 Jan-.

[8] Makary MA, Daniel M. Medical error-the third leading cause of death in the US. Bmj. 2016;**353**:i2139

[9] Adler L, Yi D, Li M, McBroom B, Hauck L, Sammer C, et al. Impact of Inpatient Harms on Hospital Finances and Patient Clinical Outcomes. Journal of patient safety. 2018;**14**(2):67-73

[10] Robertson JJ, Long B. Suffering in Silence: Medical Error and its Impact on Health Care Providers. The Journal of emergency medicine. 2018;**54**(4): 402-409

[11] Rodziewicz TL, Houseman B, Hipskind JE. Medical Error Reduction and Prevention. StatPearls. Treasure Island (FL): StatPearls Publishing Copyright © 2021, StatPearls Publishing LLC.; 2021.

[12] Committee on Diagnostic Error in Health C, Board on Health Care S, Institute of M, The National Academies of Sciences E, Medicine. In: Balogh EP, Miller BT, Ball JR, editors. Improving Diagnosis in Health Care. Washington (DC): National Academies Press (US) Copyright 2015 by the National Academy of Sciences. All rights reserved.; 2015.

[13] Singh H, Schiff GD, Graber ML, Onakpoya I, Thompson MJ. The global burden of diagnostic errors in primary care. BMJ quality & safety. 2017;**26**(6): 484-494

[14] Graber ML, Franklin N, Gordon R. Diagnostic error in internal medicine. Archives of internal medicine. 2005;**165**(13):1493-1499

[15] Meyer AN, Payne VL, Meeks DW, Rao R, Singh H. Physicians' diagnostic accuracy, confidence, and resource requests: a vignette study. JAMA internal medicine. 2013;**173**(21): 1952-1958

[16] Gandhi TK, Singh H. Reducing the Risk of Diagnostic Error in the COVID-19 Era. J Hosp Med. 2020;**15**(6):363-366

[17] Fleischmann C, Scherag A, Adhikari NK, Hartog CS, Tsaganos T, Schlattmann P, et al. Global burden of sepsis: a systematic review. Critical Care. 2015;19(1):P21.

[18] Singer M, Deutschman CS, Seymour CW, Shankar-Hari M,

Annane D, Bauer M, et al. The Third International Consensus Definitions for Sepsis and Septic Shock (Sepsis-3). Jama. 2016;**315**(8):801-810

[19] Gaieski DF, Edwards JM, Kallan MJ, Carr BG. Benchmarking the incidence and mortality of severe sepsis in the United States. Critical care medicine. 2013;**41**(5):1167-1174

[20] Torio CM AR. Healthcare Cost and Utilization Project (HCUP) Statistical Briefs. [Internet]. Rockville (MD):: Agency for Healthcare Research and Quality (US); 2006 Feb; 2013 Aug.

[21] CMS Sep-1/Sepsis Updates - 2019. 2019.

[22] Sean Townsend BD. Lemeneh Tefera. The Clinician Perspective on Sepsis Care: Early Management Bundle for Severe Sepsis/Septic Shock. 2016 Nov;**16**

[23] Rhee C, Filbin MR, Massaro AF, Bulger AL, McEachern D, Tobin KA, et al. Compliance With the National SEP-1 Quality Measure and Association With Sepsis Outcomes: A Multicenter Retrospective Cohort Study. Critical care medicine. 2018;**46**(10):1585-1591

[24] Kalantari A MH, Weingart SD. . Sepsis Definitions: The Search for Gold and What CMS Got Wrong. The Western Journal of Emergency Medicine. 2017(Aug;18(5)):951-6.

[25] Baskar R, Lee KA, Yeo R, Yeoh KW. Cancer and radiation therapy: current advances and future directions. International journal of medical sciences. 2012;**9**(3):193-199

[26] Bogdanich W. Radiation offers new cures, and ways to do harm. New York Times. 2010

[27] Keller R, Heath A. Cognitive Biases and Errors in Radiation Therapy. Radiation Therapist. 2020;29(2).

[28] Goldsworthy S, Leslie-Dakers M, Higgins S, Barnes T, Jankowska P, Dogramadzi S, et al. A Pilot Study Evaluating the Effectiveness of Dual-Registration Image-Guided Radiotherapy in Patients with Oropharyngeal Cancer. Journal of medical imaging and radiation sciences. 2017;**48**(4):377-384

[29] Caillet V, Zwan B, Briggs A, Hardcastle N, Szymura K, Prodreka A, et al. Geometric uncertainty analysis of MLC tracking for lung SABR. Physics in medicine and biology. 2020;**65**(23):235040

[30] Basu T, Goldsworthy S, Gkoutos GV. A Sentence Classification Framework to Identify Geometric Errors in Radiation Therapy from Relevant Literature. Information. 2021;**12**(4):139

[31] Weiser TG, Regenbogen SE, Thompson KD, Haynes AB, Lipsitz SR, Berry WR, et al. An estimation of the global volume of surgery: a modelling strategy based on available data. Lancet (London, England). 2008;372(9633): 139-44.

[32] Pugel AE, Simianu VV, Flum DR, Patchen DE. Use of the surgical safety checklist to improve communication and reduce complications. J Infect Public Health. 2015;**8**(3):219-225

[33] Haynes AB, Weiser TG, Berry WR, Lipsitz SR, Breizat A-HS, Dellinger EP, et al. A Surgical Safety Checklist to Reduce Morbidity and Mortality in a Global Population. New England Journal of Medicine. 2009;**360**(5):491-499

[34] Organization WH. Blood Safety and Availability 2020 [Available from: https://www.who.int/news-room/fact-sheets/detail/blood-safety-and-availability.

[35] Prevention CfDCa. Blood Safety Basics [Available from: https://www.cdc.gov/bloodsafety/basics.html.

[36] Dzik WH, Corwin H, Goodnough LT, Higgins M, Kaplan H, Murphy M, et al. Patient safety and blood transfusion: new solutions1 1The opinions expressed are those of the authors and do not represent official AABB policy. Transfusion medicine reviews. 2003;**17**(3):169-180

[37] CMS. State Operations Manual. Appendix A - Survey Protocol, Regulations and Interpretive Guidelines for Hospitals [updated 2-21-20. Available from: https://www.cms.gov/Regulations-and-Guidance/Guidance/Manuals/downloads/som107ap_a_hospitals.pdf.

[38] Bell EJ, Lutsey PL, Basu S, Cushman M, Heckbert SR, Lloyd-Jones DM, et al. Lifetime Risk of Venous Thromboembolism in Two Cohort Studies. Am J Med. 2016;129(3):339.e19-26.

[39] Lisa Baumann Kreuziger MAYYL, MD, MSc; David Garcia, MD; Mary Cushman, MD; Maria DeSancho, MD; and Jean M. Connors, MD. COVID-19 and VTE/Anticoagulation: Frequently Asked Questions. July 15, 2021 [Version 11.0; :[Available from: https://www.hematology.org/covid-19/covid-19-and-vte-anticoagulation.

[40] Henke PK, Kahn SR, Pannucci CJ, Secemksy EA, Evans NS, Khorana AA, et al. Call to Action to Prevent Venous Thromboembolism in Hospitalized Patients: A Policy Statement From the American Heart Association. Circulation. 2020;**141**(24):e914-ee31

[41] Benjamin EJ, Virani SS, Callaway CW, Chamberlain AM, Chang AR, Cheng S, et al. Heart Disease and Stroke Statistics-2018 Update: A Report From the American Heart Association. Circulation. 2018;**137**(12):e67-e492

[42] Haque M, Sartelli M, McKimm J, Abu BM. Health care-associated infections - an overview. Infection and drug resistance. 2018;**11**:2321-2333

[43] Monegro AF, Muppidi V, Regunath H. Hospital Acquired Infections. StatPearls. Treasure Island (FL): StatPearls Publishing Copyright © 2021, StatPearls Publishing LLC.; 2021.

[44] Organization. PSWH. "What is patient safety?" 2019.

[45] (CDC) CDC. Diseases and Organisms in Healthcare Settings". Healthcare Associated Infections. October 7, 2019.

[46] Voidazan S, Albu S, Toth R, Grigorescu B, Rachita A, Moldovan I. Healthcare Associated Infections-A New Pathology in Medical Practice? Int J Environ Res Public Health. 2020;17(3).

[47] Donlan RM. Biofilms and device-associated infections. Emerging infectious diseases. 2001;**7**(2):277-281

[48] Becker K, Heilmann C, Peters G. Coagulase-negative staphylococci. Clinical microbiology reviews. 2014;**27**(4):870-926

[49] (WHO). WHO. Preventing infections in health workers.

[50] (CDC) CfDC. Guidance for Unvaccinated People – How to Protect Yourself and Others." COVID-19. July 26, 2021.

[51] (CDC) C-CfDC. People with Certain Medical Conditions. May 13, 2021.

[52] (CDC). CfDC. Interim Clinical Considerations for Use of COVID-19 Vaccines Currently Authorized in the United States." Vaccines and Immunizations. . August 6, 2021.

[53] Arora HS KD, Choudhry S, Asmar BI, Abdel-Haq N. Are Stethoscopes, Coats, and Pagers

Potential Sources of Healthcare Associated Infections? Global Pediatric Health 2020;7:2333794X20969285.

[54] Currie L. Advances in Patient Safety Fall and Injury Prevention. In: Hughes RG, editor. Patient Safety and Quality: An Evidence-Based Handbook for Nurses. Rockville (MD): Agency for Healthcare Research and Quality (US); 2008.

[55] Miake-Lye IM, Hempel S, Ganz DA, Shekelle PG. Inpatient fall prevention programs as a patient safety strategy: a systematic review. Ann Intern Med. 2013;**158**(5 Pt 2):390-396

[56] Szymaniak S. Accurate falls risk assessment and interventions for preventing falls in patients in the acute care setting within a private hospital in a large capital city: a best practice implementation project. JBI database of systematic reviews and implementation reports. 2015;**13**:386-406

[57] CMS. Hospital-Acquired_ Conditions. [Available from: https://www.cms.gov/Medicare/Medicare-Fee-for-Service-Payment/HospitalAcqCond/Hospital-Acquired_Conditions.

[58] Oliver D, Healey F, Haines TP. Preventing falls and fall-related injuries in hospitals. Clinics in geriatric medicine. 2010;**26**(4):645-692

[59] Morris R, O'Riordan S. Prevention of falls in hospital. Clinical Medicine. 2017;**17**:360-362

[60] Falls prevention strategies for adult inpatients in a university hospital of Sao Paulo, Brazil: a best practice implementation project [Internet]. 2018.

[61] Cumbler EU, Simpson JR, Rosenthal LD, Likosky DJ. Inpatient falls: defining the problem and identifying possible solutions. Part I: an evidence-based review. The Neurohospitalist. 2013;**3**(3):135-143

[62] AAMC. Quality Improvement and Patient Safety Competencies Across the Learning Continuum. Washington, DC:: AAMC; 2019 [Available from: https://store.aamc.org/downloadable/download/sample/sample_id/302/.

[63] ACGME Common Program Requirements (Residency). 2018 ed2018. p. 33-6.

[64] Farley D, Zheng H, Rousi E, Leotsakos A. Field Test of the World Health Organization Multi-Professional Patient Safety Curriculum Guide. PLoS One. 2015;10(9):e0138510.

[65] IHI. Open School, Institute of Healthcare Improvement [Available from: http://www.ihi.org/education/ihiopenschool/overview/Pages/default.aspx.

[66] Training and Education Overview: ARHQ; [Available from: https://psnet.ahrq.gov/training-education.

[67] https://aamc-black.global.ssl.fastly.net/production/media/filer_public/31/13/3113ee5c-a038-4c16-89af-294a69826650/2019_update_the_complexities_of_physician_supply_and_demand_-_projections_from_2017-2032.pdf. AAMC. The complexities of physician supply and demand: projections from 2017 to 2032. . In: 2015]. HIcA, editor. 2019.

[68] Anderson M. 5 COVID-19 related medication errors reported to ISMP May 14th, 2020. Available from: https://www.beckershospitalreview.com/pharmacy/5-covid-19-related-medication-errors-reported-to-ismp.html?tmpl=component&print=1&layout=default.

[69] Kiesewetter J, Drossard S, Gaupp R, Baschnegger H, Kiesewetter I, Hoffmann S. How could the topic

patient safety be embedded in the curriculum? A recommendation by the Committee for Patient Safety and Error Management of the GMA. GMS journal for medical education. 2018;35(1): Doc15.

[70] Marx D. Patient Safety and the Just Culture. Obstetrics and gynecology clinics of North America. 2019;**46**(2):239-245

[71] Zgheib NK, Simaan JA, Sabra R. Using team-based learning to teach pharmacology to second year medical students improves student performance. Med Teach. 2010;**32**(2):130-135

[72] Boysen PG. Just Culture: A Foundation for Balanced Accountability and Patient Safety. Ochsner Journal. 2013;**13**(3):400-406

[73] Weick K, Sutcliffe K, editors. Managing the unexpected: Assuring high performance in an age of complexity2001.

[74] Team IM. Patient Engagement and Patient Safety: One and the Same Institute for Healthcare Improvement; 5 July 2017.

[75] Patient Engagement and Safety: AHRQ Agency for Healthcare Research and Quality, , ; September 2019 [Available from: https://psnet.ahrq.gov/primer/patient-engagement-and-safety.

[76] Anjana E, Sharma NAR. Jill Barr-Walker, Rachel J. Stern, Amanda K. Johnson, and Urmimala Sarkar. Patient Engagement In Health Care Safety: An Overview Of Mixed-Quality Evidence. Health Affairs. 2018;**37**(11):1813-1820

[77] Kronick R. AHRQ's Role in Improving Quality, Safety, and Health System Performance. Public Health Rep. 2016;**131**(2):229-232

[78] TeamSTEPPS® 2.0: Introduction: Agency for Healthcare Research and Quality, Rockville, MD.; March 2019 [Available from: https://www.ahrq.gov/teamstepps/instructor/introduction.html.

[79] Fiona Landgren. A guide to using data for health care quality improvement. Melbourne, Victoria.: Rural and Regional Health and Aged Care Services Division,Victorian Government Department of Human Services; June 2008. Available from: https://www.aci.health.nsw.gov.au/__data/assets/pdf_file/0006/273336/vqc-guide-to-using-data.pdf.

Chapter 3

Calling and Comradeship

Myra van den Goor and Tanya Bondarouk

Abstract

Patient safety heavily relies on doctors performing to the best of their abilities, delivering high quality of patientcare. However, changing market forces and increasing bureaucracy challenge physicians in their performance. Despite the dynamic conditions they experience, the majority performs on a high level. What exactly drives these doctors? Answering this question will shed light on how to best support doctors to be the engaged healthcare professionals that society wants and needs them to be. So patients are ensured safe and high quality of care. This chapter dips deeper into what primarily drives doctors, thus we turned to doctors themselves for answers. Being interested in their perceptions, feelings, behaviour, relations to, and interactions with, each other, this chapter relies heavily on qualitative research involving around 1000 hospital-based physicians. Conclusively, doctors can only truly blossom in an environment that stimulates their calling and that breathes a comradeship mindset, where sharing is about caring and peer-support is felt. It's alarming that these essential humanistic and relational values are supressed by today's more business-like climate in healthcare. Curtailing what primarily inspires doctors will eventually lead to doctors no longer having the time, energy and motivation to deliver the best possible patientcare. To restore the balance, we provide recommendations on the individual-, group-, and organizational level.

Keywords: healthcare quality, quality improvement, calling, humanistic values, collaborative mindset

1. Introduction

In a field as complex, dynamic, resource-intensive and with such high stakes as healthcare, physician performance is vital for delivering safe and high quality patient care. However, physicians today encounter increasing demands related to the care they feel they should give to their patients. Knowledge about what drives doctors will be helpful in optimal supporting them. So they can continue being the engaged healthcare professionals that patients need, and ensure safe and high quality of care. In this chapter we thus focus on the essence of physician performance. We share our knowledge, which is based on a thesis containing six research projects regarding this topic [1]. We unravel what drives the individual physician as well as the impact of peer-interaction on performance, motivation and well-being of the individual physician. In that context, we introduce the concepts of calling and comradeship, the essential elements of physician performance. We point out how these core values are currently threatened and provide directions of what can be done to restore the balance.

As stated above, physicians are faced with challenging tasks these days. Changing healthcare systems, changing market forces, societal pressure and increasing bureaucracy are some of these challenges [2–5]. In current literature addressing physician performance, this topic is mostly discussed on the individual level. The discourse covering performance-related aspects such as wellbeing, burnout [5–7] and poor performance [8–10] tend to be described from an individual physician perspective. We would like to point out that, in this chapter, we specifically focus on the discourse of engagement and calling, whereas we view these themes the positive counterpart of burnout. Thus, all content that is targeted at stimulating calling could therefore be framed as preventive for burnout.

Despite a focus on the individual when addressing performance, the work context, and especially peer interaction, is a known driving force for individual performance [11]. Teamwork and a collaborative mindset have increasingly become cornerstones in modern modern healthcare, with physicians increasingly performing in teams rather than individually. On top of this, effective teamwork has been explicitly linked to patient safety [12]. Thus, good interpersonal peer-relationships are essential in facilitating teamwork and the quality and safety of patientcare [11–13].

The abovementioned highlights physicians' crucial role in patient safety and the current challenges doctors face in performing to the best of their abilities. It also raises attention to performance being increasingly about teamwork, in which interpersonal connection becomes essential in the sphere of patient safety. In our overall aim to unravel the essence of physician performance, we thus explored what drives the individual physician as well as the impact of peer-interaction on performance, motivation and well-being of the individual physician. Through exploring these issues, we intended to enhance understanding of the essence of physician performance, of what makes doctors tick. Our findings indicated two overarching themes expressing the essence of physician performance: on the individual level, doctors deem calling vital to bloom. On the peer-interaction level, comradeship arose as necessary to flourish. We will briefly introduce these two concepts in this introduction and elaborate upon them in more detail in the paragraphs two and three below.

Calling, i.e. a career that provides a sense of meaning or purpose and is used to help others, emerged as an essential element. We found physicians to be highly committed and dedicated professionals with humanistic practice at the heart of their performance. A profession so strongly rooted in the fundaments of human values paves the road for a work-related sense of meaning and purpose, in turn leading to high levels of commitment, motivation and inspiration. Thus, having a calling emerged as a key component. This finding indicates that individuals only truly flourish when they feel committed and dedicated.

Comradeship, i.e. an environment were doctors feel connected, psychological safe and responsible for each other, arose as the second essential element. We found comradeship to reflect a broad feeling of a supportive group atmosphere. This indicates that relational values are essential to be at your best as an individual doctor. The findings indicate that individuals can only truly blossom in an environment that breathes a collaborative mindset, where sharing is about caring and mutual trust, and cohesion and peer-support are felt.

In paragraph four, we will outline our alarming outcome, indicating the increasing clerical burden threatening these essential values. As a result, it negatively affect doctors' motivation, empathy, well-being and performance.

Which, in turn potentially leads to a decline in the quality and safety of patientcare. This knowledge can provide us with directions in how to put physicians' core values in the spotlight, support them in their performance and thus ultimately, contribute to the safety and quality of the patient care they provide. We will point those directions out on the individual-, group-, and organizational level in more detail in paragraph five.

Before discussing these aspects, we will briefly highlight the methodological rationale of this chapter and the practical setting in which our research has taken place.

1.1 Methodological rationale

This chapter has the essence of physician performance at its heart. In an era that breathes personalized healthcare, we believe that a personalized approach fits scientific research regarding this topic. Capturing physicians' stories and exploring opinions and reflections is the foundation in understanding the essence of physician performance. Thus, we turned to doctors themselves for answers. Being interested in their perceptions, feelings, behavior, relations to, and interactions with, each other, this chapter relies heavily on qualitative research involving hospital-based physicians. We split our main goal, unravelling the essence of physician performance, into two challenges to gain a more detailed understanding of physician performance. The first challenge, containing four research projects, focusses on peer-interaction and how this interaction shapes the performance of the individual physician. Since physicians increasingly perform in teams, rather than individually, where interpersonal connection is an essential element in performing well, we argue that, in order to unravel the essence of physician performance, it is important to focus in on the peer-interaction aspect. This challenge unravels how the individual doctor is influenced (either stimulated or discouraged) by peers. The concept of comradeship arose from these research projects. The second challenge involved two research projects exploring physicians' perceptions of performance. As we were interested in the essence of physician performance, we considered it essential to explicitly bring in physicians' perceptions and experiences on this topic. This exploration exposed the concept of calling as essential element.

1.1.1 Methods

We used various methodological and analytical methods to address our challenges including: literature review of poor physician performance, review of disciplinary law verdicts, expert interviews regarding the topic poor performance, in-depth interviews addressing soft signals, surveys handling psychological safety and performance feedback, observation and in-depth interviews with a focus on the impact of peer group reflections, written reflections regarding physicians' views on their own performance and in-depth interviews unravelling physicians' perceptions on high performance. Literature search strategies followed the topics of the research projects, i.e. poor performance, soft- weak signals and performance concerns, psychological safety, reflection, professional development and multisource feedback, physician performance, high performance and professional culture. In aligning the research projects, we specifically added literature targeted at teamwork, motivation and calling. The outline below provides further information on the methodological an analytical approaches we employed, see **Figure 1**.

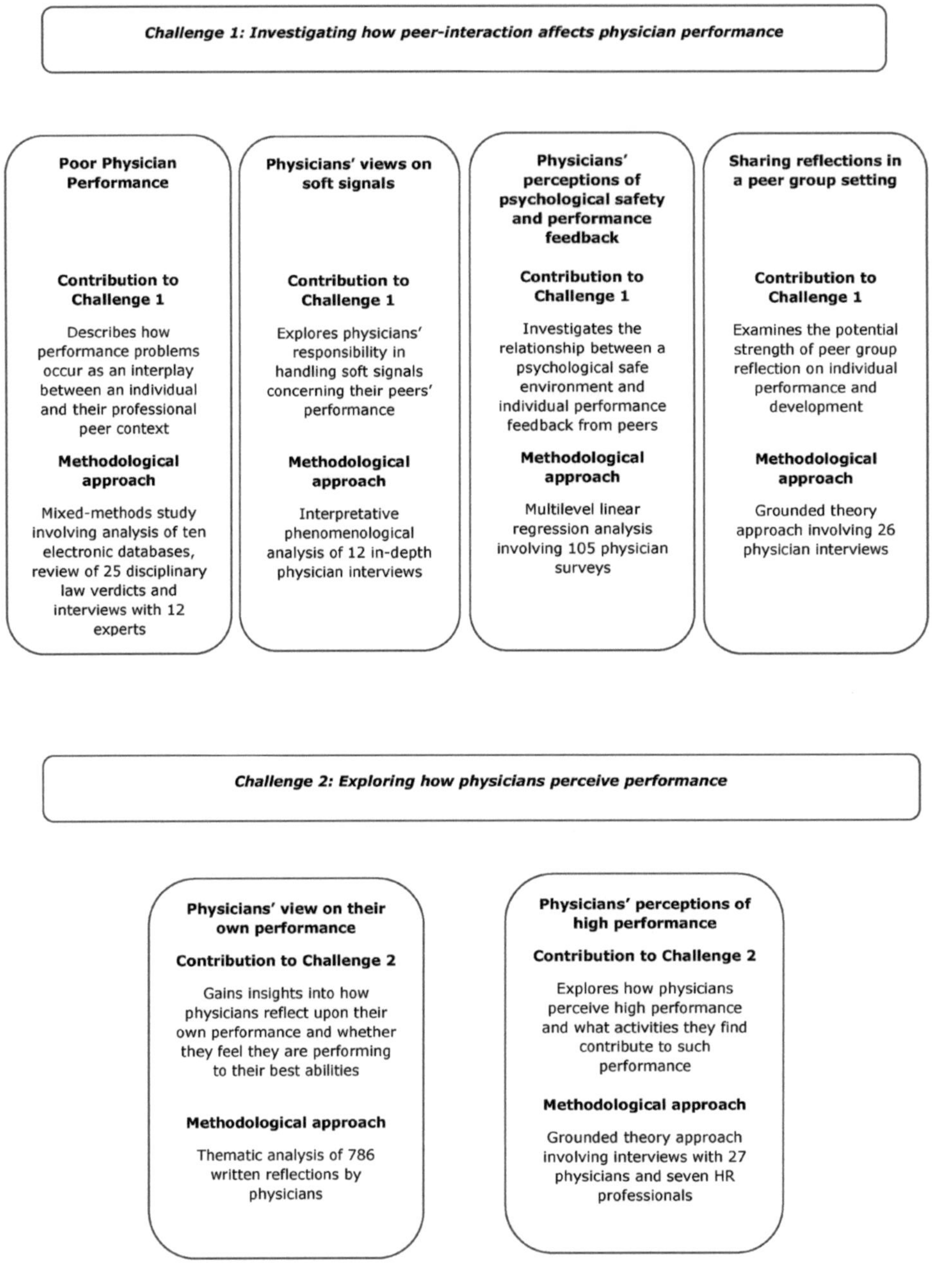

Figure 1.
Overview of the methodological and analytical approaches.

1.2 Setting the stage

This chapter is based on research taking place in the Dutch hospital setting. A characteristic in the Netherlands is the variety in physicians' employment status within the same hospital organisation. Physicians may be either employed by the hospital or organised in independent entrepreneurships. Most hospitals have both employed physician groups on the hospital's payroll and various independent entrepreneurships autonomously responsible for their "mini enterprises" within hospitals. Within a hospital, all the hospital-based physicians come under a medical board as a counterpart to the hospital board. The role of the medical board is to stand up for and maintain the interests of all physicians in their hospital, regardless of their employment status. For example, quality and performance issues are regulated by the medical board on behalf of all physicians.

2. Calling amidst physician performance

> *'Seeing patients and their families at their worst and most vulnerable moments strongly motivates me to be as emphatic and humanistic as I can be; that doesn't feel damnatory, on the contrary, it gives the uttermost satisfaction and appreciation'*

This quote from a participating physicians of the thesis reflects how doctors feel an intense dedication to their patients and consider humanistic practice at the heart of being a doctor. The overall conclusion from our findings show that physicians view the medical profession as one that provides a deep sense of meaning and purpose, where motivation and inspiration derive from their dedication to helping their patients. **Figure 2** presents a concise overview of the findings regarding calling.

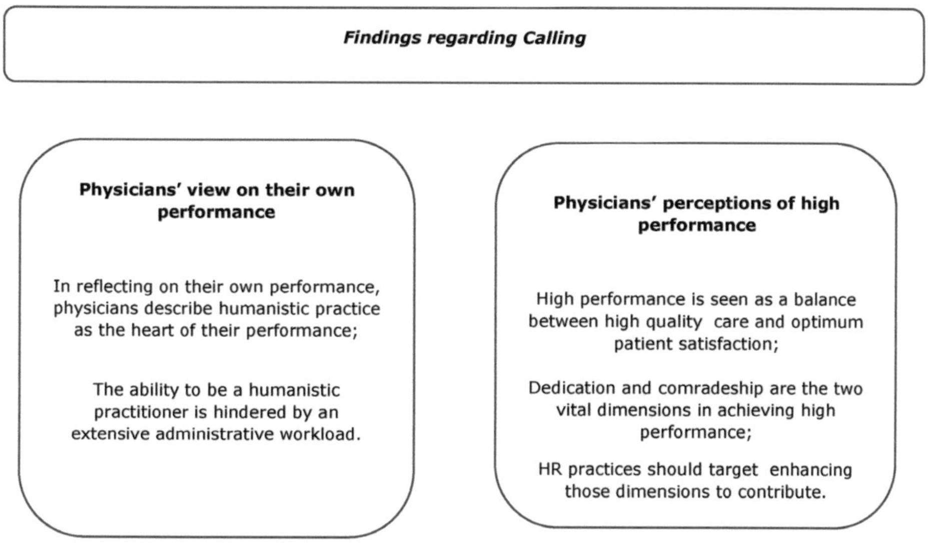

Figure 2.
Overview of the findings regarding calling.

In clarifying how we moved from performance, via motivation to calling, we will first briefly share existing knowledge on physician performance and how motivation forms a crucial element in high performance. Subsequently we will dip into motivation theories, how they differ from calling and explain the concept of having a calling.

2.1 From physician performance to motivation

> *'I'd rather not mention performance. To me, that means that you work according to an pattern or schedule. I feel that I work from engagement, not just 'perform"*
>
> *Participating physician*

The high stakes in healthcare ensure that many stakeholders become involved with, and have opinions on, the topic of 'physician performance'. These implicit ideas are made explicit in numerous charters and guidelines, all having roots extending back to the classic and oldest of all codes of conduct: the Hippocratic Oath [14, 15]. Despite the remarkable changes in medical science, the Hippocratic Oath has survived as an ideal for almost 2500 years, inspiring physicians to reinvent and uphold valued ethical principles regarding their performance [2]. It captures the core values of the medical profession, centring on the duty to help sick people and avoid harm [16].

Since healthcare is a human activity, these professional values are still considered fundamental to compassionate, ethical and patient-centred care and thus to a physician's performance [17–21]. Many documents translate these values into more hands-on guidelines and formulate good medical practice in concrete terms of knowledge, skills, communication, teamwork and maintaining trust and safety [22–24]. At the most practical level, competence frameworks describe the actual knowledge, skills and abilities that physicians should have in order to provide high quality patient care [25, 26].

Defining physician performance is complex since it encompasses all the aforementioned perspectives ranging from values to actual competences. Incorporating all these elements leads to definitions of professional performance as 'a physician committed to the health and well-being of individuals and society through ethical practice, profession-led regulation, and high personal standards of behaviour' [27]. From a more practical perspective, physician performance can be viewed as that what physicians are actually seen to do in practice, being a reflection of their adherence to values and the necessary skills and competences [28]. These definitions encompass a wide variety of aspects, ranging from values, commitment, behaviour to actual medical-technical expertise. Reflecting on knowledge of high performance in general, individual-related elements as intrinsic motivation and engagement are identified the most critical. The latter corresponds with the deep-seated dedication to their patients that physicians in our research projects exposed. Therefore we followed the path from performance to motivation in our aim to unravel the essence of physician performance.

2.2 From motivation to calling

> *'Getting to know the person behind the patient creates understanding, a deeper relationship and motivation to meet the goal for the patient'*
>
> *Participating physician*

Human motivation as a driving force of behavior and performance has been extensively studied, extending out from the realm of philosophy to the psychological, behavioral and management domains [29]. As a result, a rich variety of theories have been presented, all with their own specific angle. Well-known theories include Maslow's [30] need hierarchy theory (individual human motives are related to work), Herzberg's [31] motivation hygiene theory (hygiene factors in the context surrounding a job predict satisfaction and future motivation), Porter and Lawler's [32] expectancy theory (individual differences in abilities and skills plus role clarity link job effort to actual job performance), Locke and Latham's [33] goal setting theory (task performance is enhanced by specifying targets to achieve) and Bandura's [34] self-efficacy theory (self-confidence lies at the heart of an individual's incentive to act or to be proactive). We will briefly discuss two other theories (Self Determination Theory and Job Demands Resources Theory) in a little more detail as examples to explain how, in our research, calling was identified as the best-fitting concept for driving physician performance [35–38]. Self Determination Theory, although one of the older theories, was chosen because of its frequent citations (Ryan and Deci's [35] article has 35,697 citations according to Google Scholar) and the Job Demands Resources Theory because it is well established in the medical domain and referred to in the Vison Document of the Federation of Medical Specialists in the Netherlands [39].

According to Self Determination Theory, the nature of motivation predicts many important outcomes such as psychological health, wellbeing, deep learning and effective performance [35, 36]. Psychological health and performance benefit most from a high level of intrinsic motivation. This theory posits that three basic psychological needs (i.e. autonomy, competence and belongingness) need to be fulfilled in order to perform at one's best. In Bakker and Demerouti's Job Demands Resources Model (JD-R model), performance predictors are classified into job resources (e.g. autonomy, harmony, colleague support) and job demands such as perceived pressure, emotional demands, work-home conflict) [37, 38]. In this model, performance will blossom when the motivational process dominates, when job resources are widely available and when job demands are minimal. Where the JD-R model emphasises work-related characteristics, the Self Determination Theory puts basic psychological needs central.

> *'my heart sends me to the hospital with joy: patients and their families still touch and inspire me every single day and that's exactly what being a doctor is all about for me.'*
>
> *Participating physician*

As this quote from a participating physician expresses, none of the abovementioned motivation concepts truly fits the deep-seated dedication to their patients that doctors expressed in our research. We found that physicians' motivation and inspiration derive primarily from their dedication, and from the meaningfulness of the doctor-patient relationship [1]. An analysis of nearly 800 written reflections, targeted at physician performance, indicated that physicians experience being a humanistic practitioner at the heart of their performance. They feel that all other activities build on this humanistic practice, translated into daily practice by striving to do the best for their patients. Gaining and sharing knowledge and competences, being accountable and being transparent are means that can contribute to the best patient care. Interviewing 28 physicians and 7 HR professionals underlined the perception of a doctor as a deeply dedicated and committed professional, going that extra mile for their patients. That extra mile was even demonstrated by doctors participating in interviews after working hours, wanting to contribute to improvements, giving up their time to talk to us, despite their heavy workloads and time restraints. Their strong dedication to their patients resulted in their opinion that dedication is more than just an antecedent of high performance, as it is described in most research. They viewed dedication an essential component of high performance. We found that passion and ambition are incorporated in physicians' culture and thus shape their view of high performance. Dedication, passion, commitment and intrinsic motivation thus shape physicians' sense of meaning and purpose and drives them to perform at their best. Concepts that are all intertwined and positively related to high performance. Putting humanistic care, meaningfulness and dedication central, the concept of having a calling, i.e. having a career that provides a sense of meaning or purpose and is used to help others, best fitted the deep-seated dedication and arose as one of the two essential elements in physicians' performance [40].

2.3 Having a calling

> *'You have to be extremely motivated, to do your utmost best if patients need your care. To earn and redeem the trust that people confide in you'*
>
> *Participating physician*

Being a doctor is primarily a people business, helping others in their most vulnerable hour of need. In a profession so strongly rooted in in the fundaments of human values, a work-related sense of meaning and purpose seems self-evident. Having a meaning is assumed to influence important work-related outcomes, therefore we turn to what is known about the concept of calling [40]. Despite the growing popularity of this topic in everyday life, the literature on 'calling' is still in its infancy and only recently been seen in the medical domain [41–43]. A variety of definitions exist for 'calling' to a vocation. Dik and Duffy's seems to well reflect the general tone in defining a calling as a career that (i) involves an external summons, (ii) provides a sense of meaning or purpose, and (iii) is used to help others in some capacity [40]. The first component states that motivation comes from an external source, intentionally leaving the source undefined since this may range from God to the needs of society to serendipitous fate. The second aspect posits that one's efforts should fit into a broader framework of purpose and meaning in life; a process that is believed to help people find stability and coherence in life. The third element draws on the historic interpretation that the purpose and meaningfulness should contribute (directly or indirectly) in some positive way to "the common good" or wellbeing of society.

Freely translated from Dik & Duffy's definition, we portray calling as the sweet spot, the coinciding centre of a Venn-diagram, consisting of the following three elements: Doing what one is meant to do, Sense of purpose and meaning, and Helping others, see **Figure 3**.

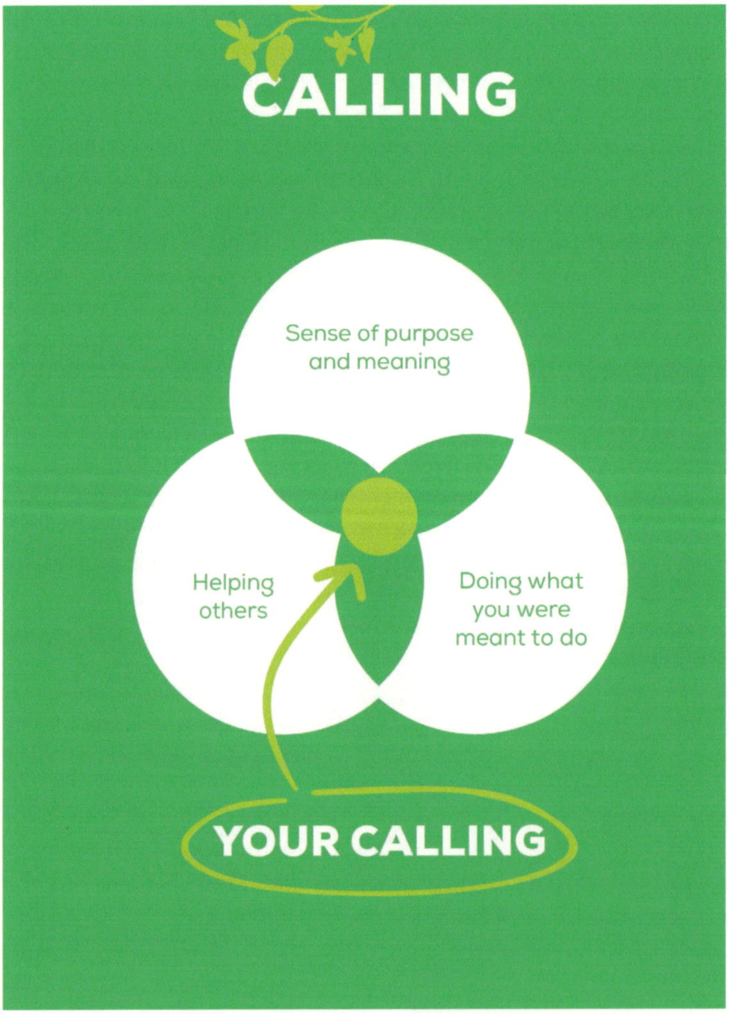

Figure 3.
Calling.

In an extended overview, Duffy and Dik conclude that, between 2007 and 2017, approximately 40 studies have been completed examining how a sense of calling links to work-related and general wellbeing outcomes, including increased career maturity, academic satisfaction, job satisfaction, career commitment, life meaning and life satisfaction [42, 44, 45]. Research in the medical domain has been limited to medical students, and indicates that first-year students feel strongly that medicine is the career they are called to, and that students interested in primary care most strongly express the presence of a calling [41]. Having a calling also bolsters medical students who have lower levels of self-efficacy and it is positively correlated with career commitment [43]. If, and how, physicians perceive this calling after graduation is still unknown. In terms of living out a calling, it is suggested that individuals actively craft their job to make it more meaningful or prosocial [46]. Despite these positive outcomes, over-investing in one's work has a potential dark side so it is advisable to ensure a healthy pursuit of any calling [42, 47]. Given the often extreme working hours and workloads of physicians, this could be a dark side to take seriously.

3. Comradeship amidst physician performance

> *'I did not expect to get emotional during the session, but it happened anyway. In my colleagues' reactions, I felt genuine interest, concern and empathy. I mean, patient contact is very important, but so is working with a group of colleagues you feel comfortable and safe with; that makes up three- quarters of your job satisfaction'.*

This statement from one of the participating physicians in the thesis, describes in a nutshell how 'comradeship' arose as one of the two overarching themes. The overall conclusion of our findings indicates that physicians perceive a safe work environment, with peers that you can trust and rely on, not only as one of the most important drivers, but as a vital dimension of optimum individual performance. **Figure 4** illustrates our findings regarding comradeship. Building on these findings, we portray comradeship as the coinciding centre of a Venn-diagram consisting of the following three elements: Feeling responsible, Feeling connected and Feeling psychological safe, as illustrated by **Figure 5**.

We will further elaborate on these three elements of comradeship below. Since comradeship emerges from team-performance, we will start by briefly setting the context of knowledge on team-performance.

3.1 From team-performance to comradeship

> *'The assurance that we have each others back, gives an enormous amount of work pleasure'*
>
> *Participating physician*

Physicians increasingly perform in teams rather than individually. When addressing team or teamwork, the general consensus in the research literature is that a team consists of two or more individuals who have specific roles, perform interdependent tasks, are adaptable and share a common goal [48]. Teamwork is the ongoing process of interaction between team members as they work together to provide care to the patients [49]. When referring to teams, we specifically mean teams of physicians. Turning to the teamwork literature, a plethora of studies highlight the benefits and importance of teamwork, and specifically in healthcare. Teamwork has been associated with a higher level of job satisfaction [50, 51], a higher quality of care [52–54], an increase in patient safety [55, 56] and greater

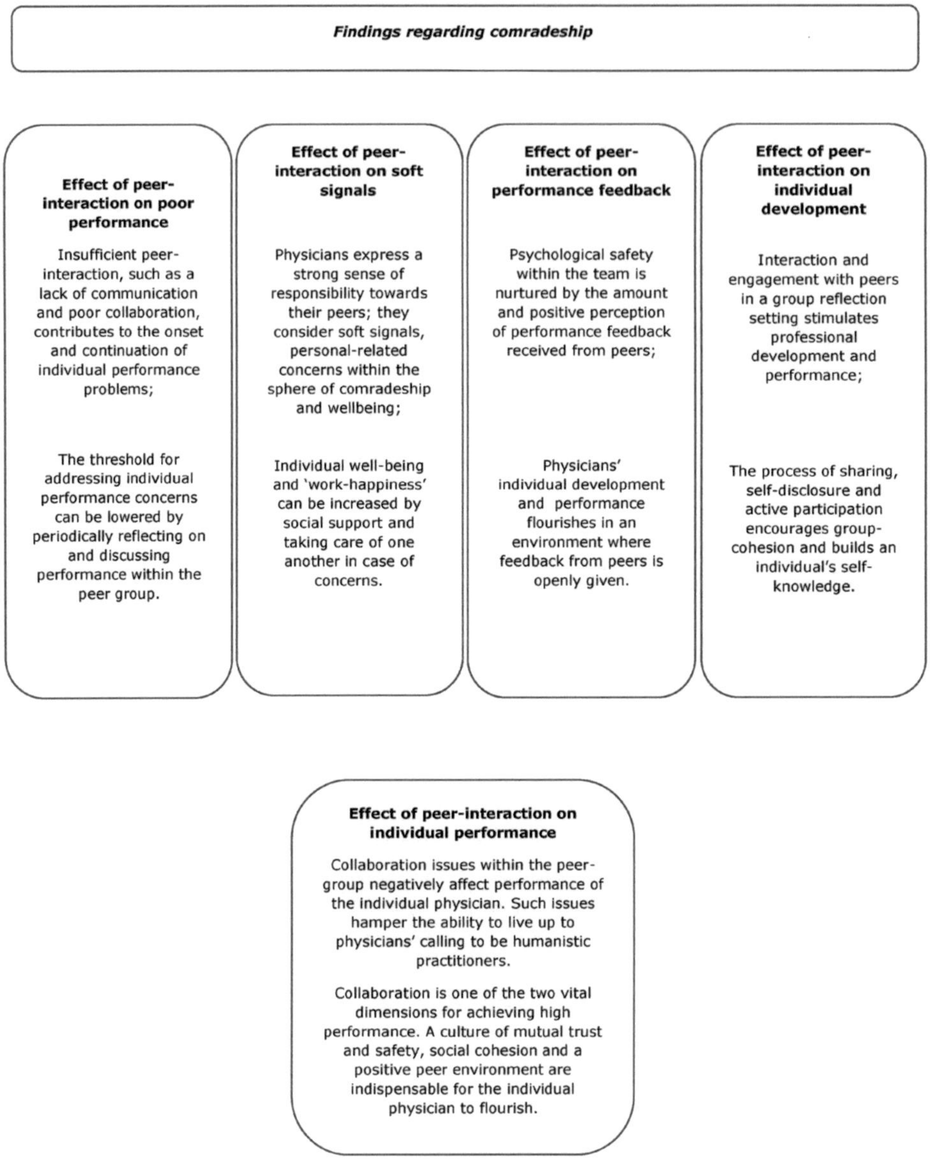

Figure 4.
Overview of the findings regarding comradeship.

patient satisfaction [57]. The extensive literature on healthcare teams has identified interpersonal-related topics including mutual respect and trust, collaboration, conflict resolution, participation and cohesion as required underpinning conditions for staff satisfaction and team effectiveness [58, 59]. Given the highly interdependent nature of physician teams, high quality peer-relationships are even more crucial in achieving high quality physician performance, both on the individual and the group level.

Turning to the current knowledge and discourses on teamwork and team performance, prior research has increasingly recognized the significance and benefits of effective teamwork in modern healthcare. Effective teamwork is linked to quality and safety of patient care because teams make fewer mistakes than individuals do [12, 60, 61]. Teamwork is also an important predictor of

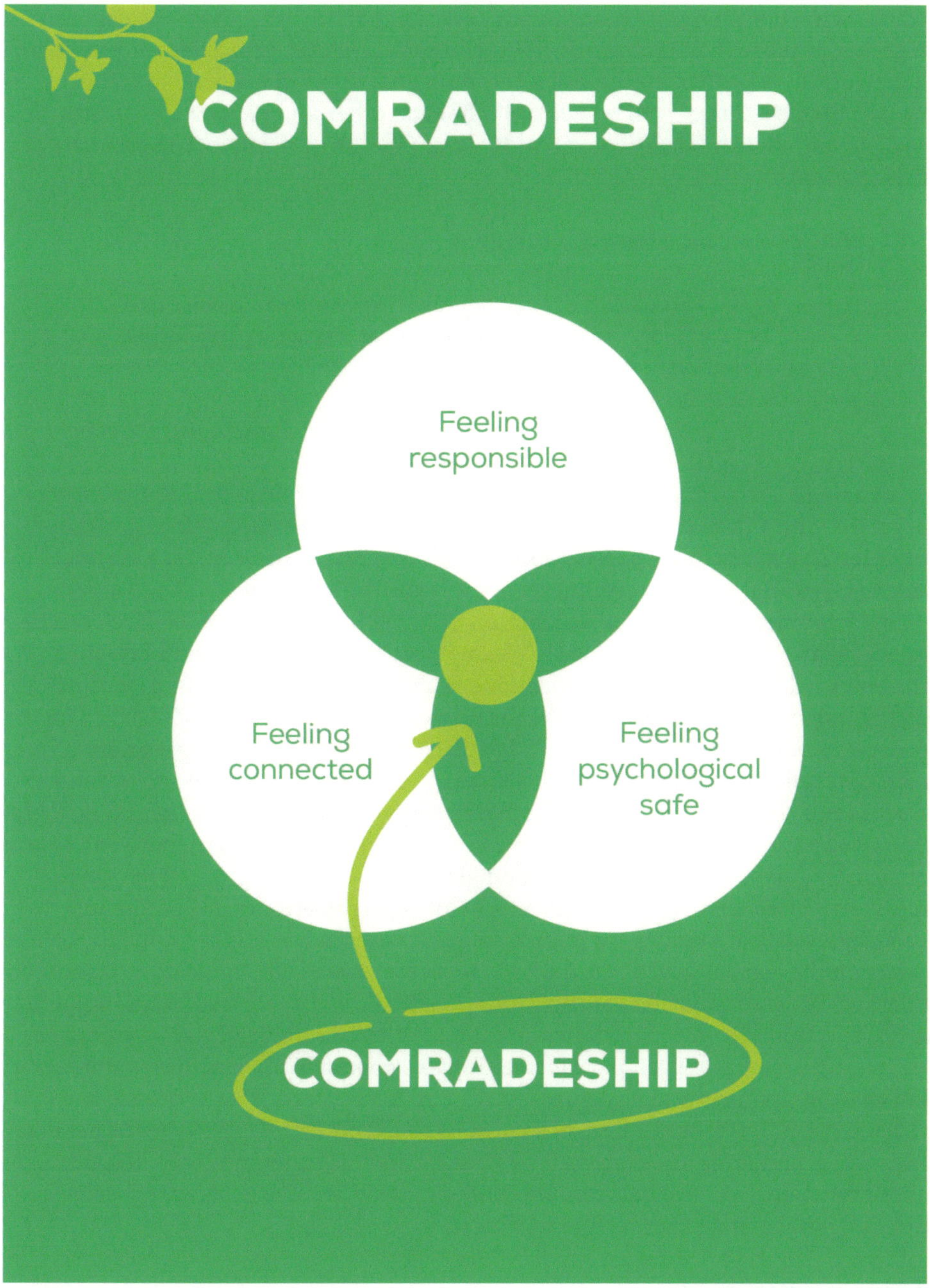

Figure 5.
Comradeship.

individual aspects such as wellbeing and job satisfaction [52]. The knowledge, skills and attitudes needed for effective teamwork include mutual performance monitoring, backup behavior, adaptability, team leadership and a team orientation [48, 60]. Psychological safety, i.e. the safety within the team to take interpersonal risks, is reported in the literature as an important aspect of high performing healthcare teams [62–64]. The importance of effective teamwork in healthcare is undisputable, affecting patient safety as well as the individual healthcare professional himself. Prior research points to a variety of conditions for effective teamwork. However, physicians in our research portray how they -ideally- work together as more than teamwork. Thus comradeship taps into a deeper level than 'just working together' to achieve a common goal. Physicians need to feel connected to one another, feel responsible for each other and psychological safe. In such a comradeship situation, individuals can bloom and deliver the best care to their patients.

3.2 Feeling connected; sharing is caring

> *'I didn't expect to get emotional, but it happened anyway. I felt a genuine interest, care and empathy in my colleagues' reactions. I mean, contact with my patients is very important, but being a member of a group were I feel comfortable makes up three quarters of my work pleasure'*
>
> *Participating physician*

Sharing builds connection within teams, whether you share knowledge, stories or reflections. Connecting fuels constructive peer-relationships, which are known to be fertile ground for the professional development and performance improvement [11]. Social support within a team increases individual well-being and even 'work-happiness' [65]. Individuals bloom in an environment were feedback can be openly shared with each other [66]. We dug deeper into this topic and investigated the potential power of sharing reflections in an peer-group setting and its effect on the individual physician [67]. We found that sharing is definitely caring. The process of sharing, self-disclosure and active participation encourages group-cohesion and also enhances individuals' self-knowledge. It offers the possibility to discuss and compare one's own and others' perceptions, gaining a nuanced insights into one's professional performance. Sharing reflections was experienced as a source of social support and deepened communal relationships on a group level. On the individual level, sharing reflections was helpful in realising actual change and creating a sense of urgency for improvement. These findings thus point to a positive effect on the team as well as the individual performance level, indicating a close correlation. Thus we conclude that performance should not be viewed on an individual level, it should always incorporate the context of this individual. As Groysberg et al. [68] observed: when a top performer leaves a company, their achievement levels fall sharply, and may still be depressed even up to five years later. It thus seems that, still too often, it is ignored that relationships shape performance alongside personal knowledge and skills. As expressed by Ramani and colleagues [69, 70], it is not about following recipes, but about investing in relationships in order to disclose, discuss, reflect on and learn from feedback.

3.3 Feeling responsible

> *'in that difficult time, I just stood by him, letting hm know that I was there for him"*
>
> *Participating physician*

Physicians express a strong sense of responsibility towards their peers, to take care of one another and look after each other. They consider it their responsibility to pick up an act on soft signals, i.e. observable deviances from a colleague's normal behaviour, appearance or communication style [65]. Physicians even consider soft signals as personal related concerns, within the sphere of well-being. As a colleague, they feel co-responsible for their peers' wellbeing: a striking example of comradeship. Prior research underscores this finding, stating that well-functioning teams can actually protect their members from the negative effects of work-related stress by enhancing occupational wellbeing indicators such as better physical and mental health [71, 72]. Our findings showed that physicians feel the need to take care of each other by actively picking up on signals or concerns and then offering a helping hand.

We considered that a situation where relations are likely to be strained, such as having a poorly performing colleague, would provide us with valuable information on how peers act and interact with one another [73]. On the interaction level, this research showed that low levels of responsibility, reflected in insufficient collaboration and a lack of addressing and speaking up amongst peers, provide fertile ground for individual performance issues to flourish and potentially develop into poor performance. This finding underscores the need to show responsibility and create a culture of speaking up and blame-free discussion of performance concerns. This echoes the literature stating that a supportive environment is necessary for effective teamwork and high team performance; an environment showing 'backup-behavior', where feedback is regularly given, poor performers are dealt with, and tough issues can be brought up [48, 75].

3.4 Feeling psychological safe

> *'hearing colleagues' struggles in an open and safe atmosphere, that offers the opportunity to be more open yourself'*
>
> *Participating physician*

The concept of psychological safety has extensively be expounded upon by Amy Edmondson and identified as the most important aspect of high performing teams [62–64, 74]. Organizational research has identified psychological safety as a critical factor in understanding phenomena such as voice, teamwork and team learning. Edmondson defines psychological safety as 'the shared beliefs that a team is safe for interpersonal risk taking and such environment exudes a sense of confidence that the team will not embarrass, reject, or punish someone for speaking up' [62]. Translated to daily practice, interpersonal risk-taking means the willingness to bring up tough issues, ask questions, seek help, admit errors, back each other or simply say 'I'm not sure, I don't know' within your team. Teams whose members feel comfortable speaking honestly with each other, even when expressing contrarian perspectives, are the teams most likely to try new things and outperform others. Specifically, a dynamic, contact-intensive and interdependent environment, such as healthcare, is likely to benefit from physicians feeling psychologically safe within their teams. Every interpersonal encounter contains a possibility to either build or destroy psychological safety, since it is really about what happens every time at that micro-level. It is in essence about questioning yourself: if I do or say this here, will I be hurt, embarrassed or criticised? A negative response indicates psychological safety and so you can proceed. This also means that actions unthinkable in one setting, can be readily taken in another owing to different beliefs about the probable interpersonal consequences. This phenomenon is called 'tacit calculus': 'the assessment of interpersonal risk associated with a given behaviour against the particular interpersonal climate' [75].

In a more tangible form, individual supportive behaviour encompasses being accessible and approachable, admitting when you do not know something, willing to show fallibility, being inclusive instead of punishing, encouraging the embracing of error and, when others cross boundaries, set in advance, and fail to perform up to these standards, holding them accountable fairly and consistently [76]. It can be argued that this interpersonal risk taking is especially important in the field of physician performance since this is a field of frequent peer-interaction under often limited time and resources combined with heavy workloads.

Physicians in our research underscore the importance of feeling psychological safe. Creating a psychologically safe environment encourages speaking up in terms of giving and receiving performance feedback [1, 66]. Performance feedback is more positively perceived by physicians who experience a higher level of psychological safety within their team. High levels of psychological safety and performance feedback are not only crucial for professional development and improving the performance of the individual physician, they also result in fewer errors and better patient outcomes [63, 77].

4. Calling and comradeship threatened.

> *'I feel that nowadays, registration rules in the hospital. That goes at the expense of my engagement and empathy and that really frustrates me'*
>
> *Participating physician*

We conclude calling and comradeship shape the essence of physician performance. That is what makes doctors tick and go that extra mile for their patients. Neuroscientific research sheds an extra light on this, explaining how the production of the happy hormone oxytocine appears to be important when it comes to connection, social contact and pleasure [78–80]. The production of oxytocine is stimulated when one has a feeling of purpose or meaningfulness. It is also stimulated in an environment of high trust. It seems that also from a neuroscientific point of view, calling and comradeship fuel work-related happiness.

That brings us to the alarming finding in our research: calling and comradeship are threatened especially by an increasing clerical burden. Although humanistic practice arises from dedication, passion and ambition, forming the heart of being a doctor, this humanistic care seems to be suppressed by today's more business-like climate in healthcare. Our findings show that increasing and heavy administrative workloads are perceived as an alarming threat to physicians' performance. This worrisome finding reflects the current era of marketisation in healthcare, shifting from people to processes, productivity and efficiency [3]. Aspects that have gained popularity in an era of declining societal trust in the medical profession due to critical incidents [81] and modern society's demands for greater transparency, accountability and measurable outcomes [82]. The doctors in our research confirmed findings elsewhere that the increasing clerical burden is leading to limited face-to-face time with patients [83]. Curtailing what primarily inspires doctors will eventually lead to doctors no longer having the time, energy and motivation to deliver the best possible care [84]. Where humanistic care is at the heart of physician performance, dedication evolves around human values such as caring, compassion and respect [21]. Doctors' dedication will therefore only flourish if the same humanity-related aspects receive adequate attention. Where Rider et al. [85] advocate reinforcing humanistic and relational aspects of care on the organizational level, we feel this should be the focus of attention on all levels, from the individual physician through to policy and society as a whole.

To place the above-mentioned call in a broader theoretical and philosophical perspective, we draw on Habermas's theory of communicative action and the parallel of the perceived discrepancy between values on one side of the spectrum and commercialization on the other side. Habermas discriminates 'lifeworld' from 'system' [86]. The 'system' consists of administrative, economic and political responsibilities and focuses on rules, checklists and costs – it is the world of money and power. Conversely, the 'lifeworld' builds on experience, everyday encounters between people, shared meaning, understanding and values – the world of shared knowledge [86, 87]. As illustrated by **Figure 6**.

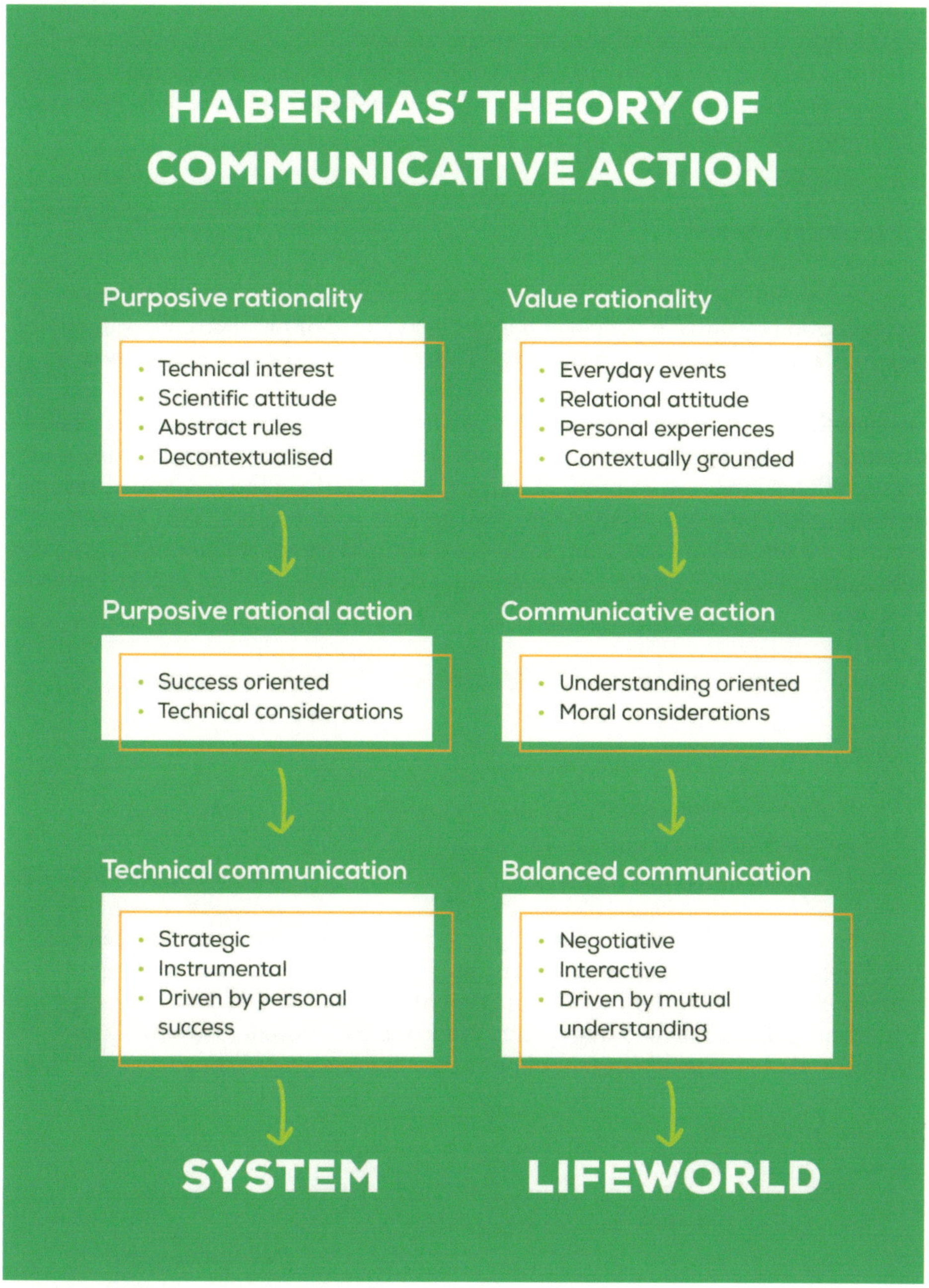

Figure 6.
Habermas' theory of communicative action.

Ideally, the values of the 'lifeworld' are conditioning, and the 'system' depends on, and follows, the 'lifeworld' with supporting rules and regulations. However, the 'system' sometimes becomes parasitic as it tends to colonize the 'lifeworld', creating a world of checklists and regulations, where values and relationships are subordinate, and regulations can become meaningless. Habermas argues that this leads to social instability since it may lead people to overlook significance or meaning. This social instability can be recognized in the healthcare arena, where the growing commercialization has resulted in a decline in medical values [20].

Related to our findings, the increasing clerical burden of the 'system' is threatening meaning and humanistic practice in the 'lifeworld'. Given that significance, meaning and purpose are all vital to physician performance, we hope that our findings contribute to the societal call for change and plea for voice to be given to physicians' 'lifeworld' [87].

5. The way forward

Based on our findings, we strongly advocate countering the climate of commercialisation by putting people in the spotlight ahead of process and productivity. By stimulating calling and comradeship. The results of our research represent a scientific argument for a broader societal call for change to 'soften' the current business-like environment that healthcare has become. Giving voice to physicians' lifeworld can and should be executed on the individual, department or group and organizational level. We will thus describe the implications and recommendations on these levels, targeted at supporting 'calling' and 'comradeship'. This appears necessary if we, as a society, want to secure dedicated professionals going that extra mile in our own hours of need when we ourselves become patients and are in need of safe care.

5.1 Recommendations for the individual level

5.1.1 Self-care

> *'because of everything that's going on in out organization, I am in a bad place. I really need do something about that, not sure what at this moment'*
>
> *Participating physician*

To be a dedicated doctor and colleague, it is crucial to take care of oneself and those around. Physicians' self-care thus should be viewed as an element of professional behaviour. As Jean Wallace described in the Lancet some years ago: "Physician wellness; the missing quality indicator [5]." Taking care of one's own physical and mental wellbeing should be a number one priority of every physician.

5.1.2 Leadership skills

> *'Professionally, we are highly trained, but we lack expertise in leadership and communications skills, those skills are simply lacking'*
>
> *Participating physician*

Our findings identified a desire in doctors for improved leadership and collaboration skills. This could be realised on an individual level in post-academic training programmes. From a leadership perspective, we found that inclusive leadership behaviour is beneficial in improving the quality of interpersonal relationships. Meaning: invite your colleagues to speak, explicitly show your appreciation, proactively ask for other opinions, offer a helping hand, reflect on an d give feedback, share and self-disclose. This can, and should, be enacted by all physicians, whether or not they have a 'formal' leadership position.

5.2 Recommendations for the department/group level

5.2.1 Invest in your team

> *'collaboration is the key, working in a pleasant team is motivating, that you really work hard together and stay in contact with each other, so our team-meetings are invaluable to me'*
>
> *Participating physician*

Individuals can only blossom within a culture of trust and safety, and therefore investing in developing such a culture seems essential, especially since the absence of psychological safety often contributes to breakdowns in collaboration [88]. Peer groups or departments can invest in comradeship by periodically collectively discuss and reflect on individual and group performance. Group reflection encourages professional development and performance, lowers the threshold for speaking up and creates an opportunity to help and advise each other. Invest as a group in discussions regarding medical topics or teambuilding activities. In addition to the work context, social activities are also important in optimising interpersonal connections. Groups and departments should in general invest in optimising group cohesion since this is known to build trust within a team.

5.2.2 Take care of each another

> *'if I have a gut feeling that something is going on, I just ask my colleague what's up and what I can do to help. Sometimes jus a cup of coffee and listening can be enough, that's what you do for each other'*
>
> *Participating physician*

Cohesion can be built through various activities especially when things did not work out as expected. Discuss adverse events, complaints or disciplinary rulings and support each other in such circumstances. Helping a colleague when they are facing an adverse event or medical error, builds fruitful relationships [89]. The impact of adverse events is intense and support form colleagues of great value [90]. When confronted with soft signals, pick up and act on them.

5.2.3 Build on the talents in your team

> *'right now it's more or less: it's your turn now, you're next. Even if that person is not really the best equipped colleague for that task. We should change this'*
>
> *Participating physician*

Teams should build on the unique talents and motivations of the individual physicians within the group since such a strength-based climate is a prerequisite for numerous positive effects and well-being [91, 92]. If a team manages to go further and ensure that members can spend at least 20% of their professional effort focused on the dimensions of work that they find most meaningful, this will dramatically lower the risk of burnout since it directly fuels ones calling [93, 94].

5.2.4 Put calling and comradeship on the agenda

> *'I'm working with these colleagues for a long time, but we never talk about our passion or how to improve as a team, that is really strange when I think about it now'*
>
> *Participating physician*

Physicians deem calling and comradeship their core values. It is astonishing that simultaneously, these values are hardly explicitly discussed within groups or departments. Meetings predominantly evolve around organizational-, patient-related-, financial-, or productivity aspects. How to stay engaged and what every team member can do to contribute to an open and safe environment deserves at least the same attention.

5.3 Recommendations for the organizational level

Given their strong links to quality of care, patient safety and patient satisfaction, having an engaged and collaborative physician workforce is critical for healthcare organisations [95, 96]. To foster dedicated doctors working in dedicated teams, healthcare organisations should invest in a collaborative mindset.

5.3.1 Facilitate groups and departments to foster calling and comradeship

> *'It would be helpful if our organization would encourage teams to reflect on individual and team-performance'*
>
> *Participating physician*

Facilitating groups and departments to optimise their group cohesion is helpful in achieving a collaborative mindset. Since the hospital board and the medical board are jointly responsible for the quality and wellbeing of their physicians, facilitating groups to spend time together and invest in their team and the individual team members should not be optional and solely a group's responsibility. On top of that, organizations could actively engage in the discourse regarding calling and comradeship; by proactively discussing these themes in team-meetings organization-wide or by organising a training or workshop.

5.3.2 Implement guidance and support

> *'you notice that people in multidisciplinary teams are very dedicated and passionate, they have a lot of knowledge and they really complement each other'*
>
> *Participating physician*

Comradeship can be enhanced by formal support or coaching programmes, investing in multidisciplinary collaboration and performance evaluations on a team level, followed by guiding and support. Physicians deal with unique challenges (such as medical errors and malpractice suits) and have a professional identity and role that is distinct from other disciplines. Because of this, fruitful peer interaction and peer support have always been part of how physicians deal with these circumstances [97]. The topic of peer support is gaining popularity and formal peer support programmes are implemented in many institutions [89]. However, the informal support aspects and interactions have become difficult given a more productivity-driven-, time- and resource effective mindset. This mindset has led to an erosion of peer support and a greater sense of isolation for many physicians [97]. In an attempt to counterbalance these eroding forces, the Mayo Clinic created dedicated meeting spaces for physicians and scientists with free fruit and beverages, computers and lunch tables. These spaces were successful in generating a sense of community and comradeship [97]. To promote engagement and satisfaction within their staff, they further funded small groups of physicians to have a meal together every other week and discuss topics that explored the virtues and challenges of being a physician. These sessions led to improvements in both meaning in work and burnout for participants [98].

5.3.3 Restore the possibility to organically spend time.

> *'We used to have a room for our entire group, so we would discuss stuff very easily between patients or so. Right now we hardly see each other'*
>
> *Participating physician*

Nowadays, it is believed that every encounter should be as 'efficient' as possible. With this side-effect of the current commercialisation of healthcare, the benefits of organically spending time together, sharing with and helping colleagues seem to be becoming overshadowed. In order to restore a healthy balance, such encounters should be re-enabled, if not organically, then through institutionalisation.

6. Conclusion

Engaged physicians working constructively in teams are prerequisite for patient safety and high quality of care. However, increasing clerical burden and limited face-to-face time with patients due to the current marketization climate in healthcare, are challenging physicians to perform to the best of their ability. Restoring the balance from processes and productivity towards people seems essential. Exploring what drives doctors fuels knowledge on how to best support these professionals. In this chapter, we explain how doctors deem two drivers essential regarding their performance: calling, i.e. a career that provides a sense of meaning or purpose and is used to help others, and comradeship, i.e. an environment were doctors feel connected, psychological safe and responsible for each other. Putting these human- and relational values in the spotlight is an active assignment for the individual physician, the group or department and the organization.

Author details

Myra van den Goor[1*] and Tanya Bondarouk[2]

1 Q3 BV, 's Hertogenbosch, The Netherlands

2 University of Twente, Enschede, The Netherlands

*Address all correspondence to: m.vandengoor@q3consult.nl

References

[1] Van den Goor M. Calling and Conradeship; unravelling the essence of physician performance [Thesis]. Enschede: Twente University; 2020.

[2] Askitopoulou H & Vgontzas AN (2017). The relevance of the Hippocratic Oath to the ethical and moral values of contemporary medicine. Part 1: The Hippocratic Oath from antiquity to modern times. European Spine Journal Oct 27. doi: 10.1007/s00586-017-5348-4. [Epub ahead of print].

[3] Bonfrer I, Figueroa JF, Zheng J et al. (2018). Impact of financial incentives on early and late adopters among US hospitals: observational study. British Medical Journal Jan 3;360:j5622. doi: 10.1136/bmj.j5622.

[4] Levey NN (2015). Medical professionalism and the future of public trust in physicians. Journal of the American Medical Association, 313(18):1827-1828.

[5] Wallace JE, Lemaire JB, Ghali WA (2009). Physician wellness: a missing quality indicator. Lancet, 374(9702):1714-1721.

[6] Hall LH, Johnson J, Watt I et al. (2016). Healthcare staff wellbeing, burnout, and patient safety: a systematic review. Plos One, 11(7): e0159015.

[7] Shanafelt, T.D., Hasan, O., Dyrbye, L.N. et al. (2015). Changes in burnout and satisfaction with work-life balance in physicians and the general US working population between 2011 and 2014. Mayo Clinic Proceedings, 90(12):1600-1613.

[8] Bismark MM, Spittal MJ, Gurrin LC et al. (2013). Identification of doctors at risk of recurrent complaints: a national study of health care complaints in Australia. British Medical Journal of Quality & Safety, 22(7):532-540.

[9] Grace ES, Wenghofer EF, Korinek EJ et al. (2014). Predictors of physician performance on competence assessments: findings from CPEP, the centre of personalized education for physicians. Academic Medicine, 89(6):912-919.

[10] Wachter RM (2012). Disciplining doctors for misconduct: character matters but so does competence. BMJ Quality & Safety, 21(12):976-978.

[11] Valentine MA, Barsade S, Edmondson AC et al. (2014). Informal Peer Interaction and Practice Type as Predictors of Physician Performance on Maintenance of Certification Examinations. Journal of the American Medical Association Surgery, 149(6):597-603.

[12] Weller J, Boyd M, Cumin D (2014). Teams, tribes and patient safety: overcoming barriers to effective teamwork in healthcare. Postgraduate Medical Journal, 90(1061):149-154.

[13] Welp A, Meijer LL, Manser T (2016). The interplay between work, clinicians' emotional exhaustion and clinician-rated patient safety: a longitudinal study. Critical Care, 20:110. DOI 10.1186/s13054-016-1282-9.

[14] Royal Dutch Medical Association (2004). Nederlandse artseneed. Available at: https://www.knmg.nl/advies-richtlijnen/knmg-publicaties/artseneed.htm

[15] Sritharan, K., Russel, G., Fritz, Z. et al. (2001). Medical Oaths and Declarations: A Declaration Marks an Explicit Commitment to Ethical Behavior. British Medical Journal, 323(7327):1440-1144.

[16] Hurwitz B & Richardson R (1997). Swearing to care: the resurgence in medical oaths. British Medical Journal, 315:1671-1674.

[17] Cassel CK, Hood V, Bauer WA (2015). A Physician Charter: The 10th Anniversary. Annals of Internal Medicine, 157(4):290-291.

[18] Lesser CS, Lucey CR, Egener B et al (2010). A Behavioral and Systems View of Professionalism. Journal of the American Medical Association, 304(24):2732-2737.

[19] Medical Professionalism Project (2002). Medical Professionalism in the new millennium: a physicians' charter. The Lancet, 359:520-522.

[20] Relman AS. (2007). Medical Professionalism in a Commercialized Health Care Market. JAMA, 298:2668-2670.

[21] Rider EA, Kurtz S, Slade S et al. (2014). The International Charter for Human Values in Healthcare: An interprofessional global collaboration to enhance values and communication in healthcare. Patient Educ Couns, 96:273-280.

[22] General Medical Council (2013). Ready for revalidation: the Good medical practice framework for appraisal and revalidation. Available at: https://www.gmc-uk.org/-/media/documents/The_Good_medical_practice_framework_for_appraisal_and_revalidation___DC5707.pdf_56235089.pdf.

[23] Medical Board of Australia (2014). Good Medical Practice: a Code of Conduct for doctors in Australia, issued March 2014.

[24] Royal Dutch Medical Association (2007). Medical Professionalism Manifesto. Available at: https://www.knmg.nl/web/file?uuid=90993000-e3b8-4713-9e8d-28a7d85eb918&owner=5c945405-d6ca-4deb-aa16-7af2088aa173&contentid=1571.

[25] Frank JR & Danoff D (2007). The CanMEDS initiative: implementing an outcomes-based framework of physician competencies. Medical Teacher, 29(7):624-647.

[26] Ten Cate, O., Snell, L., and Carracio, C. (2010). Medical competence: the interplay between individual ability and the health care environment. Medical Teacher, 32(8):669-675.

[27] Frenk J, Chen L, Bhutta ZA et al. (2010). Health professionals for a new century: transforming education to strengthen health systems in an interdependent world. Lancet, 376(9756):1923-1958.

[28] Lombarts K (2019). Physicians' Professional Performance between Time and Technology. 2010Uitgevers, Rotterdam. ISBN 978-94-90951-53-5.

[29] Steers RM, Mowday RT, Shapiro DL (2004). The future of work motivation theory. Academy of Management Review, 29(3);379-387.

[30] Maslow AH (1954). Motivation and personality. New York: Harper & Row.

[31] Herzberg, F. (1966) Work and the nature of man. Cleveland: World Publishing.

[32] Porter LW & & Lawler EE (1968). Managerial attitudes and performance. Homewood, IL: Irwin.

[33] Locke EA & Latham GP (1990). A theory of goal setting and task performance. Englewood Cliffs, NJ: Prentice-Hall.

[34] Bandura A (1977a). Self-efficacy: Toward a unifying theory of behavioral change. Psychological Review, 84: 191-215.

[35] Ryan RM & Deci EL (2000). Self-determination theory and the facilitation of intrinsic motivation,

social development, and well-being. American Psychologist, 55(1):68-78.

[36] Deci EL & Ryan RM (2008). Self-determination theory: A macrotheory of human motivation, development, and health. Canadian Psychology/ Psychologie canadienne, 49(3), 182-185.

[37] Bakker AB & Demerouti E (2007). The Job Demands-Resources model: State of the art. Journal of Managerial Psychology, 22(3):309-328.

[38] Bakker AB (2011). An evidence-based model of work-engagement. Current Directions in Psychological Science, 20(4): 265-269.

[39] Dutch Federation of Medical Specialists (2017). Vision Document Medical Specialist 2025; ambition, trust cooperation. Available at: https://www.demedischspecialist.nl/sites/default/files/FMS_visiedoc_MS2025(eng)_2017_PL_v02(lr).pdf (accessed 2017). pp. 13-14

[40] Dik BJ & Duffy RD (2009). Calling and vocation at work. The counseling psychologist, 9;37:424-45.

[41] Borges NJ, Manuel RS & Duffy RD (2013). Specialty interests and career calling to medicine among first-year medical students. Perspectives on medical education, 2:14-17.

[42] Duffy RD & Dik BJ (2013). Research on calling: What have we learned and where are we going? Journal of Vocational Behavior, 83; 428-436.

[43] Goodin JB, Duffy RD, Borges NJ et al. (2014). Medical students with low self-efficacy bolstered by a calling to their medical speciality. Perspectives on Medical Education, 3:89-100.

[44] Duffy RD, Dik BJ &Steger MF (2011). Calling and work-related outcomes: Career commitment as a mediator. Journal of Vocational Behavior, 78; 210-218.

[45] Duffy RD, England JW, Douglass RP et al. (2017). Perceiving a calling and well-being: Motivation and access to opportunity as moderators. Journal of Vocational Behavior, 98;127-137

[46] Berg JM, Dutton JE, Wrzesniewski A (2013). Job crafting and meaningful work. In B. J. Dik, Z. S. Byrne & M. F. Steger (Eds.), Purpose and meaning in the workplace, pp. 81-104. Washington, DC: American Psychological Association.

[47] Lysova EI, Jansen PGW, Khapova SN et al (2018). Examining calling as a double-edged sword for employability. Journal of Vocational Behavior, 104;261-272.

[48] Salas, E., Sims, D.E., Burke, C.S. (2005). Is there a “Big five” in teamwork? Small Group Research, 36(5),555-599.

[49] Clements D, Dault M, Priest A (2007). Effective teamwork in Healthcare: Research and Reality. Healthcare Papers, 7, 26-34

[50] Gifford BD, Zammuto RF, Goodman EA (2002). The relationship between hospital unit culture and nurses’ quality of work life. Journal of Health Care Management, 47(1), 13-25.

[51] Rafferty, A.M., Ball, J., Aiken, L.H. et al. (2001). Are teamwork and professional autonomy compatible, and do they result in improved hospital care? BMJ Quality & Safety, 10:ii32-ii37.

[52] Grumbach K & Bodenheimer T (2004). Can health care teams improve primary care practice? JAMA, 291(10):1246-1251.

[53] Mickan S, Rodger S (2000). Characteristics of effective teams: a literature review. Australian Health Review, 23(3):201-208.

[54] Wheelan SA, Burchill CN, Tilin F (2003). The link between teamwork and patients' outcomes in intensive care units. Am J Crit Care, 2(6):527-534.

[55] Firth-Couzens J (2001). Cultures for improving patient safety through learning: the role of teamwork. Qual Health Care, 10(2):26-31.

[56] Morey JC, Simon R, Jay GD et al. (2002). Error reduction and performance improvement in the emergency department through formal teamwork training: evaluation results of the Med Teams Project. Health Services Research, 37(6):1553-1581.

[57] Meterko M, Mohr DC, Young GJ (2004). Teamwork culture and patient satisfaction in hospitals. Medical Care, 42(5):492-498.

[58] Lemieux-Charles L, Mc. Guire WL (2006). What do we know about healthcare team effectiveness? A review of the literature. Medical Care Research and Review, 63(3),263-300.

[59] Thomas EJ (2011). Improving teamwork in healthcare: current approaches and the path forward. BMJ Quality & Safety, 20(8):647-650.

[60] Baker DP, Day R, Salas E (2006). Teamwork as an Essential Component of High-Reliability Organizations. Health Research and Educational Trust DOI: 10.1111/j.1475-6773.2006.00566.x

[61] Dietz AS, Pronovost PJ, Mendez-Tellez PA, et al. (2014). A systematic review of teamwork in the intensive care unit: what do we know about teamwork, team tasks, and improvement strategies? Journal of Critical Care, 29(6): 908-914.

[62] Edmondson, AC (1999). Psychological Safety and Learning Behavior in Work Teams. Administrative Science Quarterly, 44(2), 350-383.

[63] Edmondson, AC (2004). Learning from mistakes is easier said than done: group and organizational influences on the detection and correction of human error. The Journal of Applied Behavioral Science, 40(1), 66-90.

[64] Edmondson, AC (2012). Teaming: how organizations work, learn, innovate, and compete in the knowledge economy. San Fransisco, John Wiley & Sons.

[65] Van den Goor M, Silkens M, Heineman MJ, Lombarts K (2018). Investigating physicians' views on soft signals in the context of their peers' performance. Journal for Healthcare Quality, 40(5):310-317.

[66] Scheepers R, Van den Goor M, Arah OA et al (2018). Journal of Continuing Education in the Health Professions,38(4):250-254.

[67] Bindels E, Van den Goor M, Scherpbier A et al. (2020). Sharing reflections on multisource feedback in an peer group setting: (How) does it stimulate physicians' professional performance and development? Academic Medicine, accepted.

[68] Groysberg B, Nanda A and Nohria N (2004). The risky business of hiring stars. Harvard Business Review, 82(May): 92-100.

[69] Ramani S, Konings S, Ginsburg S, et al. (2018). Twelve tips to promote a feedback culture with a growth mindset: swinging the pendulum from recipes to relationships. Medical Teacher, 41(6): 625-631.

[70] Ramani S, Konings K, Ginsburg S, et al. (2019). Relationships as the backbone of feedback: exploring preceptor and resident perceptions of their behaviors during feedback conversations. Academic Medicine, published ahead of print, doi: 10.1097/ACM.0000000000002971.

[71] Sutinen R, Kivimaki M, Elovainio M et al. (2005). Associations between stress at work and attitudes towards retirement in hospital physicians. Work & Stress, 19(2):177-185.

[72] Williams BW & Flanders P (2016). Physician health and wellbeing provide challenges to patient safety and outcome quality across the careerspan. Australasian Psychiatry, 24(2):144-147.

[73] Van den Goor M, Wagner C, Lombarts K (2020). Poor physician performance in The Netherlands: Characteristics, causes and prevalence. Journal of Patient Safety, 16(1):7-13.

[74] Edmondson AC & Lei Z (2014). Psychological Safety: The History, Renaissance, and Future of an Interpersonal Construct. Annual Review of Organizational Psychology and Organizational Behavior, 1:23-24.

[75] Kramer RM & Cook KS, editors. (2004). Trust and distrust in organizations. Dilemmas and approaches. Chapter 10 Psychological Safety, Trust and Learning Organizations; a Group Level lens, 239-272.

[76] Nawaz H, Edmondson AC, Tzeng TH et al (2014). Teaming: An Approach to the Growing Complexities in Health Care: AOA critical issues. The Journal of Bone and Joint Surgery, 96(21):e184(1-7) http://dx.doi.org/10.2106/JBJS.M.01268.

[77] Leroy H, Dierynck B, Anseel F, et al. (2012). Behavioral integrity for safety, priority of safety, psychological safety, and patient safety: A team-level study. Journal of Applied Psychology, 97(6):1273.

[78] Zak PJ & Knack S (2001). Trust and growth. The Economic Journal, 111(470); 295-321.

[79] Zak PJ, Stanton AA & Ahmadi S (2007). Oxytocin Increases Generosity in Humans. PlosOne 2(11): e1128. https://doi.org/10.1371/journal.pone.0001128.

[80] Kosveld M, Heinrichs M, Zak K et al (2005). Oxytocin increases trust in humans. Nature, 435; 673-676.

[81] Blendon RJ, Benson JM, Hero JO (2014). Public trust in physicians—US medicine in international perspective. New England Journal of Medicine 371: 1570-1572.

[82] Brooks JV & Bosk CL (2012). Remaking surgical socialization: Work hour restrictions, rites of passage, and occupational identity. Social science & medicine 75: 1625-1632.

[83] Shanafelt TD, Dyrbye LN, Sinsky C, et al. (2016). Relationship Between Clerical Burden and Characteristics of the Electronic Environment With Physician Burnout and Professional Satisfaction. Mayo Clin Proc, 91(7): 836-848.

[84] Sinsky C, Colligan L, Li L et al. (2016). Allocation of Physician Time in Ambulatory Practice: A Time and Motion Study in 4 Specialties. Ann Intern Med, 165:753-760

[85] Rider EA, Gilligan MAC, Osterberg LG et al. (2018). Healthcare at the crossroads: the need to shape an organizational culture of humanistic teaching and practice. Journal of General Internal Medicine, 33(7):1092-1099.

[86] Habermas J. (1987) The theory of communicative action: Lifeworld and system: A critique of functionalist reason (Vol. 2). Boston: Beacon.

[87] Barry CA, Stevenson FA, Britten N, et al. (2001). Giving voice to the lifeworld. More humane, more effective medical care? A qualitative study of doctor–patient communication in general practice. Social science & medicine 53: 487-505.

[88] Rosenbaum L (2019). Cursed by Knowledge- Building a culture of Psychological Safety. New England Journal of Medicine, 380(8), 786-790.

[89] Hu Y, Fix ML, Hevelone ND, et al. (2012). Physicians' needs in coping with emotional stressors: the case for peer support. Arch Surg., 147(3):212-217.

[90] Verhoef LM, Weenink WJ, Winters S et al (2015). The disciplined healthcare professional: a qualitative interview study on the impact of the disciplinary process and imposed measures in the Netherlands. BMJ Open, 5:e009275. doi:10.1136/bmjopen-2015-009275.

[91] Van Woerkom M, Oerlemans W, & Bakker AB (2016). "Strengths use and work engagement: A weekly diary study." European Journal of Work and Organizational Psychology, 25(3): 384-397.

[92] Meyers MC, Kooij D, Kroon B et al. (2020). "Organizational support for strengths use, work engagement, and contextual performance: The moderating role of age." Applied Research in Quality of Life 15(2): 485-502.

[93] Shanafelt TD, West CP, Sloan JA, et al. (2009). Career fit and burnout among academic faculty. Archives of Internal Medicine, 169(10): 990-995.

[94] Horowitz CR, Suchman AL, Branch WT Jr, et al. (2003). What do doctors find meaningful about their work? Annals of Internal Medicine, 138(9):772-775.

[95] West CP, Tan AD, Habermann TM et al. (2000). Association of resident fatigue and distress with perceived medical errors. JAMA, 302(12):1294-1300.

[96] Shanafelt TD, Balch CM, Bechamps G, et al. (2010). Burnout and medical errors among American surgeons. Annals of Surgery, 251(6):995-1000.

[97] Shanafelt TD & Noseworthy JH (2017). Executive Leadership and Physician Well-being: Nine Organizational Strategies to Promote Engagement and Reduce Burnout. Mayo Clinic Proceedings, 92(1):129-146.

[98] West CP, Dyrbye LN, Satele D et al. (2015). A randomized controlled trial evaluating the effect of COMPASS (COlleagues Meeting to Promote And Sustain Satisfaction) small group sessions on physician well-being, meaning, and job satisfaction. Journal of General Internal Medicine, 30:S89.

Chapter 4

Digital Health and Healthcare Quality: A Primer on the Evolving 4th Industrial Revolution

Ahmed Umar Otokiti

Abstract

The inefficiencies of the healthcare sector continue to be a barrier to achieving the quadruple aim of healthcare quality improvement. The 4th Industrial Revolution has been characterized by rapid transformations due to information technology, data volume, ubiquity, and increased computer processing power. Despite all the promises and hopes of Digital health tools as a means of attaining healthcare quality, there remains many challenges and hurdles to overcome. This chapter describes the relationship between the 4th Industrial Revolution and healthcare quality as it relates to its impact on healthcare quality, applications, and challenges. Suggestions to stakeholders on ways of navigating these challenges are also discussed.

Keywords: digital health, health information technology, 4th industrial revolution, healthcare quality improvement, quadruple aim, artificial intelligence, ML, data science, patient safety

1. Introduction

1.1 Basic concepts of digital health and big data

1.1.1 Differentiating digital health from health informatics and E-health

Digital Health (DH) is an evolving multidisciplinary scientific field that seeks to monitor medical problems while also preventing new ones with the ultimate aim of improving the overall quality of health [1, 2]. These means of information technology can be applied through mobile health (mHealth), telehealth/telemedicine, activity trackers, personal wearables, and remote monitoring, and represent an interplay of the art and science of medicine to achieve overall improvement in health [2]. Due to its broad nature, DH is usually used interchangeably with health information technology (HIT).

Electronic-health or E-Health is characterized by an intersection of public health, medical informatics, the business of healthcare, information science, and health services to achieve better health for users [3]. The term comprises both technical aspects like hardware, software, and internet broadband and social elements centered on the way of thinking and networked global effect through information technology [3].

IntechOpen

1.1.2 Sources of big data and its contemporary drivers in healthcare

Big data refers to an enormous data set existing as either structured (organized), unstructured (unorganized), or mixed [4, 5]. These characteristics have been described as the paradigm of 4 "Vs:" volume, velocity, variety, and veracity [4, 6–8]. Generally, about 2.5 quintillion bytes of data are created every day worldwide and it is rather amazing that 90% of it was created in the past 5 years [9].

Sources of big data span a wide spectrum including posts from social media sites to sensors and navigation devices. It is a big challenge to determine the amount of data generated yearly by the healthcare industry due to the complex nature of healthcare data with heterogeneous sources and structures [10]. Healthcare data sources include electronic health record data (EHR), prescription compliance and refill rate, personal activity tracking devices, laboratory data, cell phone-based geographical monitoring, and remote telemedicine monitoring. About 500 petabytes of data were generated by electronic medical records alone in 2012 and it is expected to reach 25,000 petabytes by the end of 2020 [11]. The various methods/processes of big data analysis are referred to as analytics.

Many factors are responsible for our contemporary adoption and application of big data and DH. The greatest driving force is the dynamic state of computer power relative to it cost of acquisition rightly predicted by Moore's law. It states that computer power (in terms of speed and memory storage) will double every two years at the same price. In 1956, you would have had to pay $10 million for one gigabyte of storage. In 1981, the cost of a gigabyte was $ 300,000 and by the year 2000, it had dropped to $10. In 2010, the price of storing a gigabyte of data dropped to just 10¢ [12].

Another technology-based driver is the advent of cloud computing. This is the process of utilizing remote computer networks via the internet to manage, process, store, and manipulate data rather than utilizing the local or personal computer connected to the network. This phenomenon allowed for an exponential increase in the capacity of local computers, hence serving as a driver for the "internet of things," or the interconnectivity between various devices embedded with electronics, software, and sensors. Its ability to impact all major players in the healthcare industry, including the patient, healthcare provider, healthcare regulators, payers, and vendors, has been described as the Internet of Medical Things (IoMT) [13].

Another driver of big data application and DH is the advancement in genomic medicine and gene therapy [13]. Gene mapping and sequencing is an integral part of big data as it utilizes various bioinformatics processes for interpretation and storage.

The most important factor remains the paradigm shift in the role of the patient as a "consumer" of health services. Patients seek to better manage their health by playing active roles through information gathering on the internet and especially via social media networks [14]. One in three Americans has gone online to investigate a medical condition [15]. Another important factor is the changing demographics of the aging population and prevalence of chronic diseases leading to escalating cost of healthcare. In fact, the cost of chronic diseases accounts for up to 75% of healthcare cost in the US [16].

DH innovations have shown some promising results as a means of achieving efficient and cost effective care without compromising quality of care [17]. The mandate from regulators to shift from a volume- to value-based reimbursement model is a testament to the fact that the shift to reward quality, efficiency, and collaborative care is here to stay [18]. The incentive for hospitals to adopt meaningful use of digital technology due to the Health Information Technology for Economic and Clinical Health (HITECH) act, enacted as part of the American Recovery and Reinvestment Act of 2009 [19], resulted in widespread adoption of electronic health records system in the US.

1.2 Practical applications of data science in DH: traditional techniques, artificial intelligence, and machine learning

Data is the foundation of DH. Data science is the term used to describe the scientific study of the creation, validation, and transformation of data to create meaning [20]. It is composed of multiple disciplines like statistics, mathematics, and computer science (**Figure 1**). Data science is an overarching field that underlies many DH innovations like artificial intelligence (AI), machine learning (ML), deep learning, reinforcement learning, and data mining (**Figure 2**) [21].

ML is a sub-discipline of AI that uses algorithms to identify patterns in data, as such giving computers the ability to learn without being explicitly programmed to create predictive models based on training data and validated on test data.

Data mining refers to the discovery of patterns in large data sets with methods at the intersection of unsupervised learning, traditional statistics, and database systems [22]. Predictive analytics involves learning from historic data to predict likely future outcomes with an expressed degree of certainty. Clinical decision support (CDS) programs are systems set up to augment clinicians in their day-to-day complex decision-making processes [23].

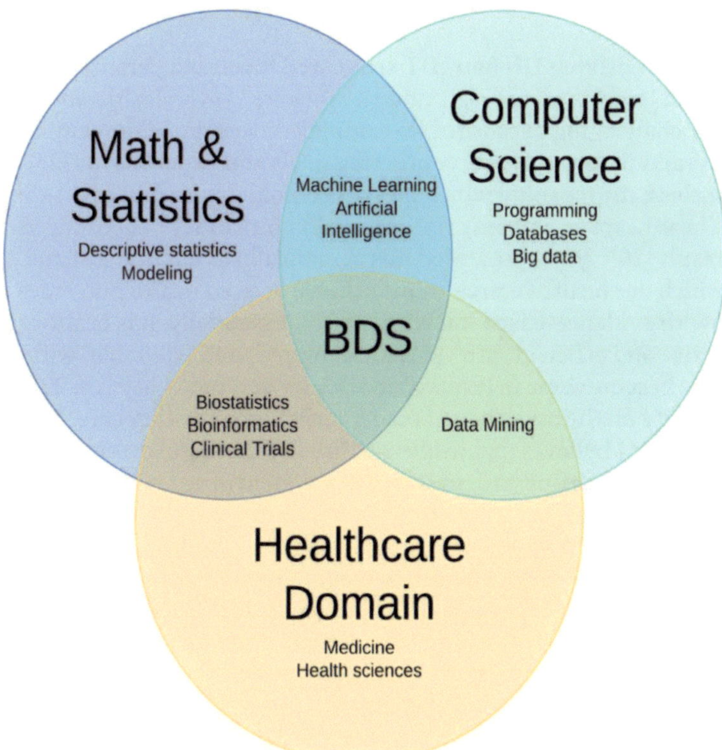

Figure 1.
Data science as a multidisciplinary field of study. Diagram reprinted with permission from Robert (Bob) Hoyt, MD, FACP, FAMIA, ABPM-CI.

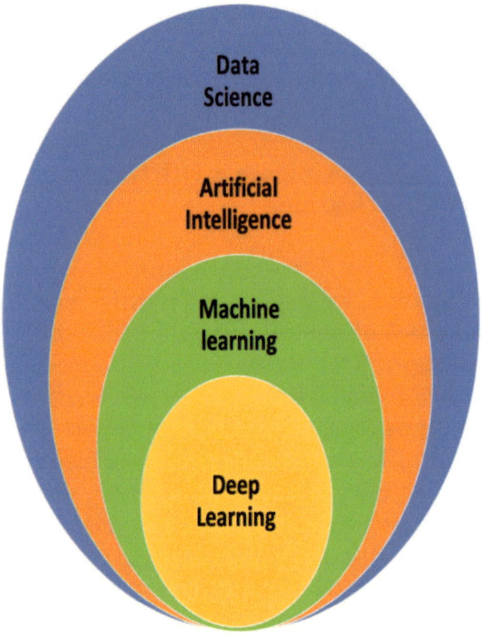

Figure 2.
Relationship between data science, artificial intelligence, and machine learning. Diagram reprinted with permission from Robert (Bob) Hoyt, MD, FACP, FAMIA, ABPM-CI.

1.3 DH's relationship with the healthcare value equation

All the factors driving DH and HIT are geared towards a paradigm shift from our present state of "sick care" to "high value healthcare" [24]. Healthcare value definition is rather challenging because of its complex ecosystem with many different stakeholders and their associated conflicting goals and expectations [25].

Nevertheless, the meaning which most stakeholders can relate to is the concept of value in healthcare as outcome (rate of quality outcome) per cost needed to achieve a result [26]. It is represented mathematically as quality/cost and is the extent to which our health interventions achieve desired health outcomes that are consistent with evidence-based knowledge [27]. Essentially, it is healthcare which is cost effective and efficient, safe, patient-centered, and equitable, with the aim of achieving the best outcome in terms of morbidity and mortality [28, 29].

Patient safety on the other hand is the foundation of quality care. The Institute of Medicine (IOM) believes that health quality is indistinguishable from Patient safety [30, 31]. I will define patient safety as a system of care delivery that prevents errors built on a culture that learns from previous mistakes. In simple terms, it is a system that functions to avoid harm to patients [32]. And healthcare quality will be analyzed in the context of the quadruple aim of quality improvement [33].

The quadruple aim is a compass to optimizing health system performance which is made up of four components: improving health outcome and experience of care, improving population health, improving healthcare cost, and improving staff engagement.

To overcome the inefficiencies of the healthcare sector in the US, healthcare organizations are encouraged to adopt methodologies like the lean or six sigma methodology that has a track record of optimizing systems in other sectors. Lean methodology involves processes put in place to reduce waste in every procedure, process, and task based on an ongoing system of improvement and learning, and focuses on eliminating waste by avoiding efforts that do not add value to the patient

[34]. Six sigma, on the other hand, is a metric-driven system used to reduce medical errors, defects, and variations in output by applying the following: design, measure, analyze, improve, and control (DMAIC) [35].

Examples of successful applications include reducing time to life saving procedure like door-to-balloon time in cardiac catherization, unnecessary antibiotics prescriptions, turnaround time for pathology reports, and clinic wait times, and streamlining electronic payment for vendors [35, 36]. Optimized symptoms that run efficiently can maximize the output of DH technologies [37].

The US spends up to 17.6% of its GDP on healthcare which is far more than that of all the other developed nations combined at 9%. Despite this amount of spending, the US ranks poorly in the World Health Organization's ranking of health system performance [38]. The public health improvement goals of the quadruple aim correspond with the goal of contemporary medicine which involves the need to achieve cost-efficient quality health through participatory and personalized medicine, ultimately ensuring optimum predictive and preventive medicine [37].

The last component of the quadruple aim is provider satisfaction and engagement. Healthcare quality can hardly be achieved without an engaged healthcare workforce. Burnout involves a state of emotional exhaustion (with or without physical fatigue) and powerlessness to change the status quo [39–41]. Up to 60% of healthcare providers experience one or more symptoms of burnout in the US [42, 43] and suicide rate amongst physicians in the US is higher than those of the general population [39]. Multiple factors are responsible for burnout which include high data and information volumes and changes in the healthcare model including a shift from volume- to value-based care [40].

Even cutting-edge EHR functionalities involving AI/ML for predictive clinical decision support are potential sources for provider dissatisfaction and burnout due to lack of regulation mandated user-centered design approach in their product development [44, 45].

1.4 The 4th industrial revolution and its peculiarities

The 4th Industrial Revolution is philosophical and ideological construct by the world economic forum which postulates on how digital, physical, and biological technology have uniquely combined together in our contemporary world creating new opportunities and challenges [41].

The first Industrial Revolution was powered by steam in the 18th century, the 2nd powered by electricity in the 19th century, and the 3rd in the 20th century powered by technology [46]. Although the 4th Industrial Revolution is considered by many as a direct extension of the 3rd, the 4th differs due to the unprecedented volume and velocity of data in addition to enhanced global interconnectivity [47].

To reap the potential benefits in the 4th Industrial Revolution, it is imperative for the healthcare sector to adopt practices like the agile methodology with the ability to "fail fast" while learning quickly in an iterative manner to achieve the desired state of healthcare quality [48].

1.5 Literature research strategy

The peer reviewed articles reviewed for this chapter were obtained from a broad literature search performed in PubMed, and Google scholar. Search terms included; "4th industrial revolution", "digital health" "quality improvement", "Digital health and patient safety", "applications of digital health for healthcare quality", "Digital health security", "Regulation of digital health". Due to the relative novelty of digital health and the 4th industrial revolution, other sources of relevant information like digital health magazines, quality improvement magazines and health informatics websites were also refer referenced.

2. Contemporary applications of HIT and DH In the context of healthcare quality improvement

The full potential of DH remains unquantifiable at this juncture mainly because of a shortage of well-conducted evaluation studies showing evidence of value added by new tools, especially those involving AI/ML [49, 50]. The rapid acceleration of DH methods and overall geometric advancement is such that any novel technology is almost outdated upon arrival. Despite all these setbacks in the application of DH, there have been some notable applications which have shown some promising results.

2.1 Individual healthcare maintenance

Remote patient monitoring involves patient data collection by appropriate providers with data either patient reported or automatically collected via apps, sensors, and any other specific gadget (glucose meters, blood pressure cuffs, or scales). This produces a vast amount of real-time data which is usually beyond the analytic capacity of the healthcare provider, creating an excellent scenario for predictive analysis of the data using ML and similar tools [51, 52].

ML analysis of bidirectional remote monitoring and EHR data has potential to provide great insights on the overall quality of individual patient care [51]. Remote monitoring has successfully been applied to diseases like congestive heart failure management (resulting in a 30% reduction in admission) [44] and diabetes management (resulting in better glycemic control compared to standard of care) [53].

2.2 Direct patient care and patient safety

Utilizing standardized risk scores and predictive analysis, some organizations have been able to predict patients that are likely to be readmitted to the hospital within 30 days after discharge [54]. Apart from the mortality benefits to the patients, the institution is also able to benefit financially as they avoid significant penalties associated with readmissions imposed by Medicare under the Medicare's Hospital Readmissions Reduction Program (HRRP) [55].

Algorithms that predict the likelihood of hospitalized patients to develop acute kidney injury during their index hospital stay have been successfully developed as well [56]. Additionally, significant reduction in sepsis mortality by algorithms leveraging the patient's data in the EHR to predict severe sepsis have also been achieved [57].

An algorithm developed using EHR data was able to predict suicide risk in individuals better than traditional clinical methods [45]. Predictive analytics tools continue to demonstrate their role in the overall reduction of in-hospital adverse events [58].

The use of CDS in antibiotics choice has been shown to significantly increase antibacterial susceptibility, thereby reducing the need for broad-spectrum antibacterial agents and the risk of antibiotic resistance [59].

Considering the complexity of cancers, the vast amount of knowledge released daily, and expansion of treatment options, the incorporation of genomic data in treatment modality all make it very challenging for clinical oncologist to choose the best personalized therapy [47]. CDS in oncology have shown some potential with assisting clinicians to navigate the challenges inherent in treatment modalities and have performed similar to multidisciplinary tumor boards [60].

The risk of failure in predictive analytics and CDS can result in significant patient harm, hence why mitigation of risk and human oversight is still an essential part of their deployment.

2.3 Healthcare operations: payment, billing, and scheduling

Predictive analytics have been used to accurately identify patients likely to skip appointments without advanced notice [61]. Additionally, they have been successfully used to anticipate peak and low utilization periods by mining previous utilization data [62]. This knowledge assists leadership in planning for changes in volume so they are ready with corresponding resources required to navigate changes in volume. Other proven applications of AI/ML include automation of invoice processing, correct coding for reimbursement, and processing of insurance denials and claims [51].

2.4 Public health essentials

The optimal state of public health of a nation should emphasize predictive and preventive care in addition to easy and equitable access to healthcare to improve overall mortality and morbidity. While the US health system falls short of these public health essentials in comparison to other developed nations, DH application has shown some promising outcomes [57].

2.5 Predictive and preventive medicine

Individual risk for developing chronic disease can be ascertained with a high degree of certainty. Integrative genetic profile has been applied successfully to determine high risk of diabetes mellitus type 2 in an individual who did not have common risk factors like obesity and family history [63].

Direct-to-consumer genetic testing for risk factors of diseases are also gaining traction with commercialized proteomic analysis testing kit for diseases like Alzheimer's disease [53]. Utilizing proteomic analysis of specific blood proteins was able to a determine if a lung nodule was benign with 90 percent accuracy during screening [64].

Similar DH based programs can assist with opioid epidemics as they have been proven to result in a 30% reduction in statewide opioid prescriptions [65–67]. Another promising application involves the development of opioid abuse risk profiles of patients using ML model and EHR data to predict patients who are prone to future abuse and overdosage [68].

2.6 Improving health access

The healthcare provider shortage coupled with the increasing aging population are factors that exacerbate healthcare access and inequity across the nation [54]. This shortage of healthcare providers and lack of access to health is worse in rural areas where 65% of non-metropolitan counties lack psychiatrists and 45% are without psychotherapists [55]. Telemedicine has shown strong evidence as a means of increasing access to mental healthcare in rural areas by providing effective treatment for mental health conditions, improving medication adherence, and effective follow up and continuity of care [69]. AI-powered chat bots can be used for initial triage based on symptoms and an expert engine can determine type and nature of visit necessary (either a virtual check-in or a face-to-face visit).

2.7 Regulations and oversight

The US Government's 21st Century Cure Act prioritized improvement in HIT, including interoperability, patient access to their health records, and improved regulatory oversight for DH [56]. As part of the Cures Act, the Food and Drug Administration (FDA) Center for Drug Evaluation and Research (CDER) has adopted analytics methodologies like "in silico" testing. This is particularly important in diseases where the smaller patient sample sizes is often a limitation of their clinical trials [70].

3. Not all that glitters is gold: challenges and shortcomings of HIT and DH utilization to achieve the quadruple aim of quality improvement

Despite the excitement which comes from the potential of DH for quality improvement, challenges exist. Not considering these challenges is akin to chasing "shiny objects" with potential for negative and adverse consequences both in the short and long term.

3.1 Overall HIT challenges across DH and big data

3.1.1 Lack of interoperability

Interoperability is the ability of different information systems to access, exchange, and cooperatively use data in a coordinated manner, within and across organizational and regional boundaries, to provide timely and seamless portability of information for optimal healthcare [57]. The healthcare data ecosystem in the US is highly fragmented with different EHR systems as a repository of patient data. These disparate EHR systems are not connected and as such their lack of interoperability is a huge set back and operational burden to DH implementation for patient safety.

3.1.2 Lack of consensus standard for evaluation and monitoring

The lack of consensus evaluation standards in DH is also a barrier to determining the value added [71]. The world of biomedical sciences is accustomed to the traditional randomized control trials as a gold standard for evaluation. Unfortunately, this is not always a practical option for most DH applications due to variation in input data and a lack of stability of deliverables needed to quantify outcomes in RCT [72]. Although various evaluation framework exists across the industry, no consensus standards have been generally accepted across board [73]. Thus, we have no standardized method of determining the effectiveness of the over 300,000 medical apps available [71].

3.1.3 Lack of emphasis on DH/hit in the context of the socio-technical impact

Most stakeholders consider DH a singular fix for the inefficiencies in healthcare [74]. But, for any DH innovation to be successful, design and implementation need to be compatible with all elements of the system engineering initiative for patient safety (SEIPS) model [75]. The elements to consider in this model include consideration of persons involved and their peculiarities, available technology and tools for success, organizational culture, type of tasks, environmental layout, care and information process/flow, and patient outcomes.

This lack of overall socio-technical consideration manifests as the absence of stakeholder input in the development of new DH tools, consequently leading to poor usability of the DH tool like the EHR, which is a significant contributor to provider burnout and inefficiency [76]. Additionally, the low usability of EHR increases the cognitive load of the healthcare provider, which contributes significantly to medical error [77].

Lack of overall consideration in the context of the socio-technical landscape increases the chances of unexpected consequences like creating workarounds in the EHR with a negative impact on patient safety [78].

3.1.4 Regulatory bodies and government unable to keep up with the dynamic changes brought on by DH

Government and regulatory agencies struggle to provide a clear-cut regulatory pathway for DH tools. Restrictions and barriers to telemedicine adoption like provider portability of license to practice across state lines, geographical restrictions, and specifics about reimbursement parity still exist and have only been temporarily lifted during the 2019–2020 COVID-19 pandemic [79]. The lack of consistent regulations of proliferating medical apps prevents a high risk to patient safety [80].

3.2 Expectations and value gaps

Innovations in most healthcare organizations in the US are driven by the need to meet basic regulatory compliance metrics and financial viability (bottom line). Healthcare leadership are more concerned about the bottom line while regulators are mostly concerned about patient safety. Patients are concerned about convenience of service and safety.

3.3 Data security and data integrity

Another important issue with DH and big data is the constant threat to healthcare data integrity and security. These occur in the form of hacking, malware, unauthorized access, and data theft. In 2019, almost 41 million medical records were affected by healthcare data breaches, mostly through hacking and ransomware attacks [81]. The average cost of these breaches to affected healthcare organizations was about $6.5million [82].

3.4 Disparity in access to DH tools

Presently, resources (infrastructure, expertise, and personnel) required to utilize DH/big data are not available to all and confer a competitive advantage to those who possess them. The resulting disparity and its consequences are contrary to the outcome we seek from DH innovations. Nearly half of the world's population do not have reliable internet access. This phenomenon is well known and described in the literature as the "digital divide" [64].

3.5 Challenges peculiar to artificial intelligence and ML

3.5.1 Lack of explainability and interpretability

Explainability describes the degree of transparency and traceability of the outcome of any AI/ML model [83]. This is particularly important because of the non-linear, highly nested structure of complex algorithms, which makes us unaware of how they arrive at their conclusion or output [65]. This characteristic, described as the "black box" phenomenon, represents a huge setback in the application of AI/ML in healthcare [66]. This is mainly due to the sensitive nature of health operations and its low tolerance for lack of transparency in decision making. Thus, those who develop AI tools must involve primary stakeholders and decision makers from the beginning to assist with transparency and adoption by end users.

3.5.2 Highly dependent on data quality and quantity

Predictive analytics and model development rely heavily on not just high volume data but also high quality data. Unfortunately, most available healthcare data are unstructured and interspersed with artifacts/"noise" which increases the chances of spurious model output even in the setting of a near-perfect model [84].

3.5.3 Prone to adversarial attacks

Adversarial attacks are either targeted or non-targeted inputs uniquely engineered to cause mis-classification and fool an AI model to produce an incorrect output [67]. This tendency for adversarial attacks in medical AI applications is due to the inherent monetary incentive for fraud in healthcare as an industry with more than three trillion-dollar annual expenditure [68]. A second reason is the technical vulnerability of the models in healthcare.

3.5.4 Implicit bias propagation

In an ethnically diverse nation like the US, an excellent AI/ML output can only be achieved if the training data utilized are equally diverse. If there is no conscious effort to ensure diversity of training data, the algorithm would be propagating the conscious and subconscious bias that exists in our society [85]. An example is an algorithm developed to detect malignant melanoma.

Malignant melanoma is treatable if detected earlier and ML algorithm can aid in early detection. However, the algorithm is at risk of bias and disparity already grounded in our society due to the lack of adequate representation of people of color/darker skin tone in training data [85]. This limitation can hinder the utility of the algorithm for people of color. Presently, most ML programs like the International Skin Imaging Collaboration Project source their training dataset mostly from fair skinned populations in the US, Australia, and Europe [85].

Other manifestations of propagated bias include: fit bits® produces inaccurate heart rate in people of color [86] and biases and mislabeling of facial recognition software with algorithm output of people of Asian descent represented as blinking facial images [69]. The risk here is the tendency to worsen all our societal ills like health disparity, inequality, gender bias, and racism, which are all hindrances to quality public health for all.

3.5.5 Unable to handle outliers/unexpected data points/events without precedence

ML algorithms are only as good as the quality of their training data set. Unexpected data points and sudden changes in pre-defined events will likely result in poor performance. This lack of initiative of the ML/AI algorithm is coupled with a lack of empathy displayed in a human-to human healthcare interaction, representing a setback for patient satisfaction.

3.5.6 Lack of consensus on disclosure of AI/ML tools in direct patient care

There exists a lot of ethical dilemmas in the application of ML tools which cannot be ignored. One of the dilemmas we face is the need for disclosure whenever ML tools are used in direct patient care [87]. In most of these applications, patients are not aware that the care from their clinician is augmented by ML algorithms even when the effectiveness of these algorithms are yet to be proven [70]. There is still no consensus amongst providers and patients alike regarding the right ethical approach to tackle this issue.

4. Separating the "wheat from the chaff:" evaluating and monitoring of HIT and DH tools for value and healthcare quality

Evaluation of DH tool/intervention is the objective and systemic assessment of a DH intervention/tool with the sole purpose of determining the efficacy, efficiency, impact, sustainability, and extent to which pre-set specific objectives are met. According to the World Health Organization, "evaluation asks whether the DH tool/project is doing the right things, while monitoring asks whether the DH tool/project is doing things right." [88]. Although monitoring and evaluation (M&E) are distinct entities, they are usually addressed simultaneously from pre-prototype/prototype stage through the pilot and demonstration/display of tool up to the stage of scale up.

4.1 Stages of monitoring and evaluation

The first stage of M&E is to identify the stage of maturity of the tool. This determination will play into the methodology/framework utilized for M&E.

After identifying the stage of maturity of tool, the next step would be to ascertain concrete baseline expectations of the tool and define appropriate claims based on stage of maturity of the DH tool. The usability of the tool is an important measure that should be evaluated in all the stages of maturity from early to late stages. It is also important to set expectations in relation to time to deliverables to guide M&E activities. A tool being developed to shorten wait time at the clinic should get input from patients about their pain points while setting M&E standards.

The next steps is to define the M&E framework to guide the process. There are well-established frameworks for M&E published in the literature; however, I favor structures that are result oriented [73, 88]. To strengthen the evaluation framework, it should be developed through a stakeholder consultative process and reviewed as needed during the life cycle of the project.

The next step is to determine who will be carrying out these M&E activities, how many resources will be required, and the time-based deliverables expected from the team in charge.

5. Navigating the challenges of HIT and DH for quality improvement: a call to action for all stakeholders

Considering the degree of rapid transformation and dynamism we are experiencing with the 4th Industrial Revolution, only organizations positioned to adapt will succeed. This adaptation requires that all stakeholders learn new skill sets as we navigate this transformation.

5.1 Stakeholder specific suggestions to navigate 4th industrial revolution

5.1.1 Government and regulatory agencies

Government regulatory oversight teams are needed to craft rules/policies to regulate broad DH principles like security, privacy/disclosures of DH tools, fairness and equity of implementation, and avoidance of bias in implementation. The regulatory rigors placed before approval of DH tools should be based on the level of risk of a DH tool in the event of failure, determined by a baseline failure mode and effect analysis.

Government mandates should ensure that DH tools maintain a well laid out process for human oversight of implementation no matter how "perfect" the tool may be.

5.1.2 Professional expert organizations

Professional organizations can assist with navigating complexities as it relates to specific requirements for M&E of DH tools developed for their subsections. Once general overall policies are established by the government or regulatory agencies to address fundamental societal issues to ensure quality and safety of DH, expert organizations can help narrow down these policies to suit their subsection of the healthcare ecosystem.

5.1.3 Payers

Payers are responsible for processing patient eligibility, enrollment, claims, and payment of healthcare services. In the US, payers exists as either governmental (Medicare/Medicaid) or private entities. A testament to the fragmented nature of the US healthcare system is the fact it has more than 900 healthcare payers as of 2020 [89]. These entities have a significant influence on how healthcare is delivered in the US based on their reimbursement schemes. As part of their basis for reimbursement of any healthcare service which has been augmented by DH, they should mandate standardized M&E of the tools to justify compensation; it is equally important to be wary of mandates that would stifle innovation.

5.1.4 Vendors

Healthcare vendors ranging from device and pharmaceutical manufacturers to core HIT and analytics developers and entrepreneurs are numerous; in fact, there are more than 370 HIT-specific vendors in the US as of 2020 [90]. Vendors also have a role to play in ensuring that DH tools do not only offer novelty but also have an in-built yardstick for evaluating their comparative effectiveness for objective assessment of their overall impact upon implementation.

5.1.5 Direct patient care organizations

Considering that these centers are the avenue for implementation of most DH tools, they must insist on implementing DH tools with a track record of adding value to patient safety and improving healthcare quality. In the event the DH tool intended for use is novel with no track record, the organization should demand a concrete basis and claims for M&E. This will assist with an objective comparison of the impact of a new tool with the status quo.

5.1.6 Healthcare providers

Healthcare providers are often laggards and usually conservative in the adoption of new tools, as consequences of failure are very high with regards to patient safety [91]. Nevertheless, the 4th Industrial Revolution permeates all sectors of healthcare and healthcare providers are directly impacted. They must actively learn how to become an information specialist and ask the right questions about a potential DH tool to be implemented [92]. Considering that they will be utilizing these tools to make important decisions about patients and their safety, it is important they are well equipped with the knowledge of how to evaluate and monitor the DH tools for optimal healthcare quality.

5.1.7 Patients and caregivers

Patients and caregivers are the ultimate intended beneficiaries of DH tools, as any failure of DH tool implemented will have an adverse consequence on their safety and quality of health [93]. In this new dispensation, they must prompt their healthcare providers to ask the right questions from the DH tools' developers. Patients and caregivers should understand that, as we progress further into the 4th Industrial Revolution, these DH tools will increasingly play an essential role in decisions about their care directly or indirectly.

6. Conclusion

The quadruple aim describes healthcare value as improved health outcomes, increase patient satisfaction, reduced costs, and healthcare provider satisfaction/ fulfillment. DH tools have shown potential in improving healthcare quality and achieving the quadruple aim, such as promoting behaviors like healthy eating and smoking cessation, improving outcome in people with chronic conditions like cardiovascular diseases, and increasing health access through telemedicine and remote monitoring [72, 94].

Although there are demonstrated impact of DH tools in healthcare quality, it is still not an overall fix able to transition us from our state of sick care to optimum healthcare quality alone. Its applications and implementation are filled with many limitations presently hindering the achievement of its full potential in healthcare quality improvement. We cannot figure out how effective a tool is without a pre-defined basis on how to ascertain its effectiveness. Presently the evaluation and performance measurement in healthcare is costly, redundant, and labyrinthine [78].

DH tools are only part of the solution and not an ultimate solution. As such every DH tool implementation should be considered in the context of the overall socio-technical ecosystem. All innovations should be based on stakeholders' input right from the start of conception. No matter how effective a piece of technology is, if it is implemented in a poorly optimized system, it will likely result in failure.

Navigating the 4th Industrial Revolution requires that all stakeholders play an active role in this transition. No doubt it brings forth many possibilities for healthcare quality improvement; however, in the absence of evaluation standards and a systematic approach to its implementation, we risk being immersed in hype born out of the hope of an elusive better outcome. DH tools are key components in achieving value in healthcare, but it is not the destination and neither is it the goal, but rather a catalyst in the process of obtaining the ultimate goal of the quadruple aim.

Conflict of interest

The author declares no conflict of interest.

Appendix 1: glossary of abbreviations

Abbreviation	Meaning
DH	Digital Health
mHealth	Mobile Health
HIT	Health Information Technology
IoMT	Internet of Medical Things
HITECH	Health Information Technology for Economic and Clinical Health
ML	Machine learning
AI	Artificial Intelligence
DMAIC	Design, Measure, Analyze, Improve, and Control
GDP	Gross Domestic Product
HER	Electronic Health Record
HRRP	Medicare's Hospital Readmissions Reduction Program
CDS	Clinical Decision Support
FDA	Food and Drug Administration
M&E	Monitoring and Evaluation

Author details

Ahmed Umar Otokiti
Department of Medicine and Clinical Informatics Group, Icahn School of Medicine at Mount Sinai, Mount Sinai Health System, 1 Gustave L. Levy Place, New York, NY 10029, USA

*Address all correspondence to: ahmedotoks@yahoo.com

References

[1] Khillar S. Difference Between Digital Health and Health Informatics 2020 [Available from: http://www.differencebetween.net/technology/difference-between-digital-health-and-health-informatics/.

[2] Zhang S, Liao R, Alpert JS, Kong J, Spetzger U, Milia P, et al. Digital medicine: Emergence, definition, scope, and future. Digital Medicine. 2018;4(1):1.

[3] Eysenbach G. What is e-health? J Med Internet Res. 2001;3(2):E20.

[4] Kruse CS, Goswamy R, Raval Y, Marawi S. Challenges and Opportunities of Big Data in Health Care: A Systematic Review. JMIR medical informatics. 2016;4(4):e38.

[5] Wang W, Krishnan E. Big data and clinicians: a review on the state of the science. JMIR medical informatics. 2014;2(1):e1.

[6] McAfee A, Brynjolfsson E. Big data: the management revolution. Harvard business review. 2012;90(10):60-6, 8, 128.

[7] Heudecker N. Hype Cycle for Big Data, 2013 2013 [Available from: https://www.gartner.com/doc/2574616/hype-cycle-big-data-.

[8] Kayyali B, Knott D, Kuiken S. The big-data revolution in US health care: Accelerating value and innovation 2013 [Available from: https://digitalstrategy.nl/wp-content/uploads/E2-2013.

[9] IBM. Bringing big data to the enterprise 2016 [Available from: https://www-01.ibm.com/software/data/bigdata/what-is-big-data.html.

[10] LeSueur D. 5 Reasons Healthcare Data Is Unique and Difficult to Measure 2016 [Available from: https://www.healthcatalyst.com/5-reasons-healthcare-data-is-difficult-to-measure.

[11] Feldman B, Martin EM, Skotnes T. Big Data in HealthcareHype and Hope 2012 [Available from: https://www.ghdonline.org/uploads/big-data-in-healthcare_B_Kaplan_2012.pdf.

[12] Cullis P. The Personalized Medicine Revolution: Greystone; 2015.

[13] Dimitrov DV. Medical Internet of Things and Big Data in Healthcare. Healthcare informatics research. 2016;22(3):156-63.

[14] Flores M, Glusman G, Brogaard K, Price ND, Hood L. P4 medicine: how systems medicine will transform the healthcare sector and society. Personalized medicine. 2013;10(6):565-76.

[15] Fox S, Duggan M. One in three American adults have gone online to figure out a medical condition: Pew Research Center; 2013 [Available from: http://www.pewinternet.org/2013/01/15/health-online-2013/.

[16] The National Academies of Sciences E, Medicine,,. Best Care at Lower Cost: The Path to Continuously Learning Health Care in America 2012 [Available from: http://www.nationalacademies.org/hmd/Reports/2012/Best-Care-at-Lower-Cost-The-Path-to-Continuously-Learning-Health-Care-in-America.aspx.

[17] Buntin MB, Burke MF, Hoaglin MC, Blumenthal D. The benefits of health information technology: a review of the recent literature shows predominantly positive results. Health affairs. 2011;30(3):464-71.

[18] Putera I. Redefining Health: Implication for Value-Based Healthcare Reform. Cureus. 2017;9(3):e1067-e.

[19] HHS. HITECH Act Enforcement Interim Final Rule 2013 [Available from: HITECH Act Enforcement Interim Final Rule.

[20] Hoyt R, editor Machine Learning Basics for Informatics Professionals. AMIA Clinical Informatics Conference; 2020 May, 20: AMerican Medical Informatics Association.

[21] West M. Acing the Machine Learning Engineering Interview 2020 [Available from: https://www.udemy.com/course/acing-the-machine-learning-engineering-interview/.

[22] Hand DJ, Adams NM. Data Mining. Wiley StatsRef: Statistics Reference Online. 2014:1-7.

[23] Sutton RT, Pincock D, Baumgart DC, Sadowski DC, Fedorak RN, Kroeker KI. An overview of clinical decision support systems: benefits, risks, and strategies for success. NPJ Digital Medicine. 2020;3(1):1-10.

[24] Fani Marvasti F, Stafford RS. From sick care to health care--reengineering prevention into the U.S. system. The New England journal of medicine. 2012;367(10):889-91.

[25] i-scoop.eu. Digital health – a matter of access, priorities, people, integration and proven value 2019 [Available from: https://www.i-scoop.eu/digital-transformation/healthcare-digital-health/.

[26] Porter ME. What is value in health care? N Engl J Med. 2010;363(26):2477-81.

[27] Lohr KN. Medicare: a strategy for quality assurance, volume I: National Academies Press; 1990.

[28] Lohr KN. Outcome measurement: concepts and questions. Inquiry. 1988;25(1):37-50.

[29] Hughes R. Patient safety and quality: An evidence-based handbook for nurses: Agency for Healthcare Research and Quality Rockville, MD; 2008.

[30] Mitchell PH. Defining patient safety and quality care. Patient safety and quality: An evidence-based handbook for nurses: Agency for Healthcare Research and Quality (US); 2008.

[31] Erickson SM, Wolcott J, Corrigan JM, Aspden P. Patient safety: achieving a new standard for care: National Academies Press; 2003.

[32] Clancy CM, Farquhar MB, Sharp BAC. Patient safety in nursing practice. Journal of nursing care quality. 2005;20(3):193-7.

[33] Bodenheimer T, Sinsky C. From triple to quadruple aim: care of the patient requires care of the provider. The Annals of Family Medicine. 2014;12(6):573-6.

[34] Catalyst N. What Is Lean Healthcare? NEJM Catalyst. 2018.

[35] Chassin MR. Is health care ready for Six Sigma quality? The Milbank Quarterly. 1998;76(4):565-91.

[36] Aminu M. Six Sigma in Healthcare: Concept, Benefits and Examples 2018 [Available from: https://draminu.com/six-sigma-in-healthcare/.

[37] Mummadi S, Pai RK, Hahn P. The Big Picture about 'Big Data'. Physician leadership journal. 2017;4(2):22-4.

[38] Starr P. Remedy and Reaction: The Peculiar American Struggle over Health Care Reform: Yale University Press.

[39] Schernhammer ES, Colditz GA. Suicide rates among physicians: a quantitative and gender assessment (meta-analysis). American Journal of Psychiatry. 2004;161(12):2295-302.

[40] Rothenberger DA. Physician Burnout and Well-Being: A Systematic Review and Framework for Action. Dis *Colon rectum*. 2017;60(6):567-76.

[41] Marr B. The 4th Industrial Revolution is here-are you ready. Forbes August Available online: https://www forbes com/sites/bernardmarr/2018/08/13/the-4th-industrial-revolution-is-here-are-youready. 2018.

[42] Jones GM, Roe NA, Louden L, Tubbs CR. Factors Associated With Burnout Among US Hospital Clinical Pharmacy Practitioners: Results of a Nationwide Pilot Survey. Hosp Pharm. 2017;52(11):742-51.

[43] West CP, Dyrbye LN, Shanafelt TD. Physician burnout: contributors, consequences and solutions. J Intern Med. 2018;283(6):516-29.

[44] Freitag TB, Taylor G, Wick L, Cunningham J, Alexy T. Novel Remote Patient Monitoring System Improves Key Outcomes. Journal of Cardiac Failure. 2019;25(8):S104.

[45] Simon GE, Johnson E, Lawrence JM, Rossom RC, Ahmedani B, Lynch FL, et al. Predicting suicide attempts and suicide deaths following outpatient visits using electronic health records. American Journal of Psychiatry. 2018;175(10):951-60.

[46] Khan G, Isreb D. 1,2,3... Here comes the 4th Industrial Revolution: PWC; 2020 [Available from: https://www.digitalpulse.pwc.com.au/fourth-industrial-revolution-guide/.

[47] Kent J. Clinical Decision Support from Dana-Farber Powers Cancer Care 2018 [Available from: https://healthitanalytics.com/news/clinical-decision-support-from-dana-farber-powers-cancer-care.

[48] Tolf S, Nyström ME, Tishelman C, Brommels M, Hansson J. Agile, a guiding principle for health care improvement? International journal of health care quality assurance. 2015.

[49] Adler P, Falk C, Friedler SA, Nix T, Rybeck G, Scheidegger C, et al. Auditing black-box models for indirect influence. Knowledge and Information Systems. 2018;54(1):95-122.

[50] Vellido A. Societal Issues Concerning the Application of Artificial Intelligence in Medicine. Kidney Dis (Basel). 2019;5(1):11-7.

[51] Davenport T. New York-Presbyterian, WorkFusion, And The Intelligent Automation Of Health Care Administration 2019 [Available from: https://www.forbes.com/sites/tomdavenport/2019/09/15/new-york-presbyterian-workfusion-and-the-intelligent-automation-of-health-care-administration/#2b0269d07e77.

[52] Choucair B, Bhatt J, Mansour R. How cities are using analytics to improve public health. Harv Bus Rev. 2014.

[53] 23and Me. About Us 2017 [Available from: https://www.23andme.com/genetic-science/.

[54] Kirch DG, Petelle K. Addressing the physician shortage: the peril of ignoring demography. JAMA : the journal of the American Medical Association. 2017;317(19):1947-8.

[55] Andrilla CHA, Patterson DG, Garberson LA, Coulthard C, Larson EH. Geographic variation in the supply of selected behavioral health providers. American Journal of Preventive Medicine. 2018;54(6):S199-S207.

[56] Gabay M. 21st Century Cures Act. Hospital pharmacy. 2017;52(4):264-5.

[57] Stoltenberg Consulting. Stoltenberg Consulting's Health IT Industry Outlook

Survey reveals six key leadership trends for 2019 2019 [Available from: https://www.globenewswire.com/news-release/2019/03/20/1757828/0/en/Stoltenberg-Consulting-s-Health-IT-Industry-Outlook-Survey-reveals-six-key-leadership-trends-for-2019.html.

[58] Lin Y-K, Fang X. First, Do No Harm: Predictive Analytics to Reduce In-Hospital Adverse Events. Available at SSRN 3273203. 2018.

[59] Anooj P. Clinical decision support system: Risk level prediction of heart disease using weighted fuzzy rules. Journal of King Saud University-Computer and Information Sciences. 2012;24(1):27-40.

[60] Sesen MB, Peake MD, Banares-Alcantara R, Tse D, Kadir T, Stanley R, et al. Lung cancer assistant: a hybrid clinical decision support application for lung cancer care. Journal of The Royal Society Interface. 2014;11(98):20140534.

[61] Ding X, Gellad ZF, Mather III C, Barth P, Poon EG, Newman M, et al. Designing risk prediction models for ambulatory no-shows across different specialties and clinics. Journal of the American Medical Informatics Association. 2018;25(8):924-30.

[62] Bresnick J. How Big Data Analytics Can Improve Patient Utilization Rates 2016 [Available from: https://healthitanalytics.com/news/how-big-data-analytics-can-improve-patient-utilization-rates.

[63] Cohen J. Examining His Own Body, Stanford Geneticist Stops Diabetes in Its Tracks: Science Magazine; 2012 [Available from: http://www.sciencemag.org/news/2012/03/examining-his-own-body-stanford-geneticist-stops-diabetes-its-tracks.

[64] Makri A. Bridging the digital divide in health care. The Lancet Digital Health. 2019;1(5):e204-e5.

[65] Samek W, Wiegand T, Müller K-R. Explainable artificial intelligence: Understanding, visualizing and interpreting deep learning models. arXiv preprint arXiv:170808296. 2017.

[66] London AJ. Artificial Intelligence and Black-Box Medical Decisions: Accuracy versus Explainability. Hastings Cent Rep. 2019;49(1):15-21.

[67] Finlayson SG, Chung HW, Kohane IS, Beam AL. Adversarial attacks against medical deep learning systems. arXiv preprint arXiv:180405296. 2018.

[68] CMS.gov. National Health Expenditures 2017 Highlights 2018 [Available from: https://www.cms.gov/research-statistics-data-and-systems/statistics-trends-and-reports/nationalhealthexpenddata/downloads/highlights.pdf.

[69] Crowford K. Artificial Intelligence's White Guy Problem 2016 [Available from: https://www.nytimes.com/2016/06/26/opinion/sunday/artificial-intelligences-white-guy-problem.html.

[70] Robbins R, Brodwin E. An invisible hand: Patients aren't being told about the AI systems advising their care 2020 [Available from: https://www.statnews.com/2020/07/15/artificial-intelligence-patient-consent-hospitals/.

[71] Gordon WJ, Landman A, Zhang H, Bates DW. Beyond validation: getting health apps into clinical practice. NPJ Digital Medicine. 2020;3(1):1-6.

[72] Murray E, Hekler EB, Andersson G, Collins LM, Doherty A, Hollis C, et al. Evaluating Digital Health Interventions: Key Questions and Approaches. American journal of preventive medicine. 2016;51(5):843-51.

[73] Kowatsch T, Otto L, Harperink S, Cotti A, Schlieter H. A design and

evaluation framework for digital health interventions. it-Information Technology. 2019;61(5-6):253-63.

[74] Li J. A Sociotechnical Approach to Evaluating the Impact of ICT on Clinical Care Environments. Open Med Inform J. 2010;4:202-5.

[75] Carayon P, Schoofs Hundt A, Karsh BT, Gurses AP, Alvarado CJ, Smith M, et al. Work system design for patient safety: the SEIPS model. Qual Saf Health Care. 2006;15 Suppl 1(Suppl 1):i50-8.

[76] Kroth PJ, Morioka-Douglas N, Veres S, Pollock K, Babbott S, Poplau S, et al. The electronic elephant in the room: Physicians and the electronic health record. JAMIA Open. 2018;1(1):49-56.

[77] Burgess DJ. Are providers more likely to contribute to healthcare disparities under high levels of cognitive load? How features of the healthcare setting may lead to biases in medical decision making. Med Decis Making. 2010;30(2):246-57.

[78] Mutter JB, Liaw W, Moore MA, Etz RS, Howe A, Bazemore *A. core* principles to improve primary care quality management. The Journal of the American Board of Family Medicine. 2018;31(6):931-40.

[79] Weigel G, Ramaswamy A, Sobel L. Opportunities and barriers for telemedicine in the US during the COVID-19 emergency and beyond. Washington, DC: Kaiser Family Foundation, May. 2020;11.

[80] Levine DM, Co Z, Newmark LP, Groisser AR, Holmgren AJ, Haas JS, et al. Design and testing of a mobile health application rating tool. NPJ Digital Medicine. 2020;3(1):1-7.

[81] Landi H. Number of patient records breached nearly triples in 2019 2019 [Available from: https://www.fiercehealthcare.com/tech/number-patient-records-breached-2019-almost-tripled-from-2018-as-healthcare-faces-new-threats.

[82] Landi H. Healthcare data breaches cost an average $6.5M: report 2019 [Available from: https://www.fiercehealthcare.com/tech/healthcare-data-breach-costs-average-6-45m-60-higher-than-other-industries-report.

[83] Holzinger A, Langs G, Denk H, Zatloukal K, Müller H. Causability and explainability of artificial intelligence in medicine. *Wiley Interdiscip Rev Data Min Knowl Discov*. 2019;9(4):e1312.

[84] Weiskopf NG, Bakken S, Hripcsak G, Weng C. A Data Quality Assessment Guideline for Electronic Health Record Data Reuse. EGEMS (Wash DC). 2017;5(1):14.

[85] Adamson AS, Smith A. Machine learning and health care disparities in dermatology. JAMA dermatology. 2018;154(11):1247-8.

[86] Piazena H, Meffert H, Uebelhack R. Spectral Remittance and Transmittance of Visible and Infrared-A Radiation in Human Skin-Comparison Between in vivo Measurements and Model Calculations. Photochem Photobiol. 2017;93(6):1449-61.

[87] Cohen IG. Informed Consent and Medical Artificial Intelligence: What to Tell the Patient? Geo LJ. 2019;108:1425.

[88] Organization WH. Monitoring and evaluating digital health interventions: a practical guide to conducting research and assessment. 2016.

[89] Price S. Largest Health Insurance Companies of 2020 – Over 370 Entries 2020 [Available from: https://www.valuepenguin.com/largest-health-insurance-companies.

[90] Health IT skills. Healthcare IT/Software Companies 2020 – Over 370 Entries 2020 [Available from:

https://healthcareitskills.com/healthcare-it-software-companies/.

[91] Hodgkins M, Khoury C, Katz C, Lloyd S, Barron M. Health Care Industry Requires A Roadmap To Accelerate The Impact Of Digital Health Innovations 2018 [Available from: https://www.healthaffairs.org/do/10.1377/hblog20180606.523635/full/.

[92] Jha S, Topol EJ. Adapting to artificial intelligence: radiologists and pathologists as information specialists. JAMA : the journal of the American Medical Association. 2016;316(22):2353-4.

[93] FDA. The FDA Recommends Only Using Cleared or Approved Medical Devices to Help Assess or Diagnose a Head Injury, Including Concussion: FDA Safety Communication 2019 [Available from: https://www.fda.gov/medical-devices/safety-communications/fda-recommends-only-using-cleared-or-approved-medical-devices-help-assess-or-diagnose-head-injury.

[94] Bashshur RL, Shannon GW, Bashshur N, Yellowlees PM. The Empirical Evidence for Telemedicine Interventions in Mental Disorders. Telemed J E Health. 2016;22(2):87-113.

Chapter 5

The Role of the Radiation Safety Officer in Patient Safety

Thomas L. Morgan and Sandy Konerth

Abstract

The role of the Radiation Safety Officer (RSO) is to prevent unnecessary exposure to ionizing radiation and maintain necessary exposures as low as reasonably achievable (ALARA). The RSO is delegated broad authority throughout the organization by senior management. This authority includes permission to stop unsafe practices and identifying radiation protection problems, initiating, recommending, or providing corrective actions and verifying implementation of these actions. For the most part, these efforts are focused on maintaining radiation doses to employees and the public ALARA. Regulations do not address a role for the RSO in reducing radiation exposure to patients, except when unnecessary exposure is suspected due to equipment malfunction or human error. There is increasing concern about the risks of cancer and other effects from the use of medical imaging procedures. This chapter will discuss the tools and resources available to the RSO to educate members of the medical community and senior management on the need to manage radiation doses to patients so that the physician is able to obtain information necessary to properly diagnose and treat patients while avoiding unnecessary exposure.

Keywords: ALARA for patients, radiation safety, justification, optimization

1. Introduction

Patients are exposed to ionizing radiation from individual radiographic or nuclear medicine procedures and from multiple procedures. In 1987, the National Council on Radiation Protection and Measurements (NCRP) published a report that evaluated the radiation doses to the U.S. population from all sources of ionizing radiation [1]. Report No. 93 estimated the annual dose to an individual at 3.6 mSv. The amount caused by medical diagnostic x-rays and nuclear medicine procedures was estimated at 0.53 mSv or 14.7% of the total dose. Doses from computed tomography (CT) scans were not listed separately. In 2006, an updated report, No. 160, estimated the average annual dose at 6.2 mSv [2]. Doses from medical procedures increased 5.7-fold to 3.0 mSv or 48.4% of the total exposure. CT scans were responsible for 1.47 mSv or 24% of the total dose. This was based on an estimated 62 million CT procedures and a U.S. population of 300 million. Doses from ubiquitous natural sources remained largely unchanged – 3.0 mSv in Report No. 93 and 3.1 mSv in Report No. 160. In 2019, a follow-on report, No. 184, evaluated medical radiation exposure alone. For 2016, an estimated 74 million CT procedures (20% increase from 2006) in a population of 323 million resulted in an average dose that was essentially unchanged from 2006–1.4 to 1.5 mSv [3]. However, the report noted an overall decrease in the average medical exposure from 3.0 mSv in 2006 to 2.2 to

2.3 mSv, due largely to a 68% decrease in dose from nuclear medicine procedures, a 25% decrease from diagnostic radiography and fluoroscopy procedures and a 39% decrease from cardiac interventional fluoroscopy procedures. These reductions were due to a variety of factors, including increased patient, physician, and manufacturer awareness (CT scans), changes in the standards of practice resulting in fewer nuclear medicine procedures and changes in technology (replacement of film-screen units to digital receptors in radiography) and standards of practice (fluoroscopy).

Several studies have chronicled the utilization of radiographic and nuclear medicine procedures in detail. For example, a retrospective cohort study of 952,420 nonelderly patients enrolled in healthcare plans across five U.S. health care markets for three years (2005 through 2007) was conducted to evaluate the pattern and source of radiation exposure [4]. Analysis of utilization data found that 68.8% (655,613) underwent at least one imaging procedure during this time frame. A total of more than 3.44 million imaging procedures were associated with these enrollees. Nuclear medicine myocardial profusion studies accounted for more than 22% of the total radiation dose to this population and CTs of the chest, abdomen, and pelvis accounted for almost 38%. CT scans and nuclear medicine procedures accounted for only 21% of the procedures but were responsible for 75.4% of the total dose to the population. Plain radiographs made up 71.4% of the procedures but accounted for only 10.6% of the total dose. More than 80% (81.8%) of the dose was delivered in an outpatient setting, most often in physicians' offices. As a second example, a study of patients admitted to a level 1 trauma facility found 10,504 radiographic studies were performed on 465 patients who suffered spinal injuries [5]. A total of 6,720 X-ray studies and 3,606 CT scans were performed which translates to an average of 14.5 X-ray studies and 7.75 CT scans per admitted patient.

Neither of these studies criticized the decisions to refer the patients for medical imaging studies. However, in the case of the utilization review study, the authors commented "that in some patients worrisome radiation doses from imaging procedures can accumulate over time underscores the need improve their use." In the second study, the authors expressed concern about cumulative radiation exposure. They urged colleagues to "be astutely aware of the implications of different imaging studies and weigh these against the benefits when ordering any study".

Elsewhere in the medical literature, there is increasing concern expressed about the potential risks of exposing patients to ionizing radiation from medical imaging procedures. In 1994, the United States Food and Drug Administration published an advisory notice to physicians and other health care professionals about serious x-ray-induced injuries to the skin from fluoroscopically guided radiographic procedures [6]. This advisory listed the types of procedures that often involve extended fluoroscopy time (e.g., 50 to 60 minutes or more) that could cause injury and discussed ways to minimize the risk of injury.

Computed tomography (CT) scanners became commercially available in 1972 and their use quickly took off. In 2000, attention was called to the potential increased lifetime risk of cancer mortality attributable to radiation from CT scan use in children [7]. More recently, in 2012 and 2013, two large retrospective cohort studies evaluated the risk of cancer from CT scans delivered in childhood and adolescence. The first study reviewed results from more than 175,000 patients scanned from 1985 to 2002 in Great Britain. For patients who received a cumulative dose of at least 30 mGy, the risk of leukemia was increased 3.18-fold; for brain cancer the risk was increased 2.82-fold for patients whose cumulative dose was 50 to 74 mGy [8]. The second study assessed the cancer risk in more than 680,000 patients, aged 0 to 19 years, who received a CT scan from 1985 to 2005 in Australia. The overall cancer risk was 24% greater for exposed versus unexposed people, after accounting for age, sex, and date of birth [9].

2. Methodology

This chapter is intended as a literature review. Search parameters included: medical indications for imaging procedures, hazards and risks of radiation exposure, risk analysis, responsibilities of a Radiation Safety Officer (RSO), laws and regulations governing use of radiation, industry best practices for prescribing medical imaging procedures. The author used his more than 25 years of experience in radiation protection to guide this search.

3. Concepts

The following concepts and principles are presented in this chapter:

Concept	Principle	Responsibility
Identify high dose imaging procedures	Risk analysis	RSO, medical physicists
Reduce radiation exposure	Justify imaging procedure; optimize dose	Referring provider, medical physicists
Educate providers on best practices	Identify and provide resources	RSO
Change practices	Implement best practices	RSO, providers, management

4. The Radiation Safety Officer

The RSO is charged with the responsibility to monitor and/or estimate the radiation exposure of staff, visitors, and the public from the use of ionizing radiation sources within the facility. In the U.S., Federal and State regulations require that these doses be maintained below certain maximum limits. From a safety perspective, best practices suggest that the RSO should take action to achieve and maintain doses as low as reasonably achievable (ALARA). This concept has been adopted as a regulatory requirement. As defined by the U.S. Nuclear Regulatory Commission (NRC) in Title 10 Code of Federal Regulation Section 20.1003 [10], ALARA means

> *"making every reasonable effort to maintain exposures to ionizing radiation as far below the dose limits as practical, consistent with the purpose for which the licensed activity is undertaken, taking into account the state of technology, the economics of improvements in relation to state of technology, the economics of improvements in relation to benefits to the public health and safety, and other societal and socioeconomic considerations, and in relation to utilization of nuclear energy and licensed materials in the public interest."*

While NRC regulations focus only on the use of radioactive materials ("licensed materials" above), state agencies that regulate the use of x-ray-generating equipment have incorporated the NRC ALARA policy and dose limits into their own radiation protection regulations.

However, neither federal nor state regulations address or require ALARA principles be applied to patients undergoing medical imaging procedures. At best, these regulations require the equipment be inspected to ensure it is operating in compliance with regulations, manufacturers' recommendations and best industry practices. In addition, the RSO is required investigate unnecessary or excessive exposures to determine the root cause and provide corrective and preventative actions to reduce or eliminate the risk of similar event.

These practices, while appropriate, are reactive, not proactive. They do not mandate a process of risk management – i.e., identifying, monitoring, and managing potential risks in order to minimize the negative impact they may have on patients.

The usefulness of medical imaging procedures is not in dispute. Clearly, an accurate diagnosis that leads to appropriate treatment outweighs the low risks of cancer or injury. However, given the large number of procedures carried out each year, a patient advocate is needed. This advocate will educate medical providers and management about the risks of excessive radiation exposure, identify areas or procedures within the organization where the potential for high doses to patients exists, and provide oversight of a process to apply ALARA principles medical imaging.

It can be argued that while the RSO is one of many individuals in a healthcare organization who have roles to play in the responsible use of these modalities, the RSO has a unique mission—that of leading the healthcare team in maintaining radiation doses ALARA. This allows for a different perspective than the provider who orders the imaging studies, the radiologic technologist who performs the studies, or the medical physicist who ensures the equipment is performing properly.

The RSO has broad responsibility for ensuring the organization achieves and maintains compliance with applicable laws, regulations and standards. This requires in-depth knowledge of equipment, personnel, facilities and operating procedures. It also requires the RSO to develop and maintain collaborative relationships with senior medical and non-medical managers as well as line managers and where feasible, the individuals who are responsible for operating the imaging equipment. Thus, the RSO is in a position bring together important stakeholders to focus efforts on reducing patient radiation doses. This puts the RSO in a unique position to become the patient advocate or to be part of the patient advocate team.

5. ALARA concepts

The principles of ALARA introduced above are based on three fundamental concepts: justification, optimization, and dose limits [11]. Justification means doing more good than harm. The benefit to the exposed individual exceeds the detriment the radiation dose causes. If the procedure is justified, it should be optimized and performed to maximize the good over the harm. Finally, the use of dose limits implies an adequate standard of protection, even for the most highly exposed individual. These three concepts will be discussed in Sections 7.1 and 7.2 below.

6. Risk analysis

Risk analysis is a prospective, structured method for assessing the likelihood of an adverse event occurring. This is followed by the design of a new procedure or modification of an existing procedure to reduce the likelihood [12]. Briefly, the process involves identifying the hazards (i.e., what could go wrong) and estimating the risk of the hazard occurring. This process requires a deep dive into policies, procedures, and equipment performance at the institution.

For the purposes of this discussion, the major hazard to be evaluated is radiation dose to patients during medical imaging procedures.

The RSO should be aware of those areas within the institution where there is potential for high radiation exposures. The hazards and risks will change and scale as the size and complexity of the institution increases. Taking a risk-informed approach, the RSO can survey the various medical imaging departments or areas to become informed about the type and number of procedures routinely performed. This will allow the RSO to focus efforts on the highest risk areas first.

Radiation dose is governed by several factors. First, the radiation output of an X-ray tube is determined by beam energy (applied voltage) (kVp), applied current (mA) and beam on time. The output is typically preset by computer, based on patient size, weight and scan length in case of plain radiographs and CT scans. With fluoroscopy, the output is determined automatically by a computer, based on the ability of the X rays to penetrate the patient. In these cases, the RSO's efforts can be focused on directing providers to educational resources that identify appropriate procedure(s) for a given medical condition and training fluoroscopy users on how to properly operate the fluoroscopy unit to achieve a good quality image at an appropriate dose.

Some patients have complex medical conditions that require fluoroscopy for both diagnosis and treatment. In these cases, a fluoroscopically guided interventional (FGI) procedure is indicated. These procedures have the potential to deliver high doses to localized areas of the skin. However, due to the diverse nature of these procedures, variation in patient size and anatomy, and other confounding factors, it is not possible set a standard technique or beam-on time. Reductions in patient doses can be achieved through specialized operator training and machine settings as described in Section 7.2.2.3 below.

Second, for nuclear medicine and nuclear cardiology procedures, radiation dose is a function of the type and amount of the radiopharmaceutical administered to the patient. The amounts are usually standardized for each radiopharmaceutical and procedure, although some may vary based on the patient's weight. There are four major hazards: administration (i) to the wrong patient; (ii) of the wrong radiopharmaceutical; (iii) in the wrong amount; or (iv) by the wrong route.

7. Policies and procedures for the RSO

Once the RSO has cataloged the institution's hazards, the next step is to prioritize dose reduction efforts. For example, an outpatient clinic or urgent care center may have only one or a few X-ray machines and perform studies limited to plain films of the head and neck, torso and extremities. In this case, the RSO's focus would be on ensuring the equipment is functioning properly, personnel are properly licensed and trained, standard imaging protocols are used, and patient identification procedures are in place to prevent unnecessary exposures (i.e., wrong patient or wrong site imaged).

In a hospital setting, the imaging needs, equipment, and modalities offered can range from a small facility with only X-ray imaging equipment, including CT scanners to a large regional medical or teaching hospital center that provides the full spectrum of imaging modalities from X-ray machines, portable fluoroscopy units, nuclear medicine and nuclear cardiology cameras, and complex fixed fluoroscopy units in the interventional radiology and cardiology areas.

In the small hospital, the RSO's efforts would be similar to the outpatient clinic example above, with the additional need to monitor CT protocols (see below). In a large hospital setting, the risk of high doses increases substantially because of the number and complexity of the cases. In this case, the RSO risk analysis efforts should be focusing on evaluating the patient workload, number and general types of procedures performed, and the state of training, certification and credentialling of the personnel involved in the imaging procedures. In general, the highest radiation doses occur in the following departments/areas [4]: nuclear cardiology, radiology, interventional cardiology, nuclear medicine, positron emission tomography (PET)/CT scans.

Patient dose reduction efforts begin with developing and implementing policies and procedures based on the three basic principles of ALARA described in Section 5 above.

7.1 Justifying imaging procedures

7.1.1 Appropriateness criteria

In the United States, the Protecting Access to Medicare Act (PARMA) of 2014 established a new program to increase the rate of appropriate advanced diagnostic imaging services provided to Medicare beneficiaries [13]. Examples of such advanced imaging services include CT, PET, nuclear medicine, and magnetic resonance imaging (MRI).

Under this program, at the time a provider orders an advanced diagnostic imaging service for a Medicare beneficiary, he/she, or clinical staff acting under his/her direction, will be required to consult a qualified Clinical Decision Support Mechanism (CDSM). CDSMs are electronic portals through which appropriate use criteria (AUC) can be accessed. This program is set to be fully implemented on January 1, 2022.

The American College of Radiology (ACR), the Society of Nuclear Medicine and Molecular Imaging (SNMMI), and the American Society of Nuclear Cardiology (ASNC) have published evidence-based guidelines to assist providers in making appropriate imaging or treatment decisions for specific clinical conditions [14–16].

Consulting and applying the AUC will help reduce the number of inappropriate and duplicative medical imaging studies ordered, thus reducing radiation dose to patients and staff if fluoroscopy is used. The role of the RSO in this process would be to educate providers about this resource and the upcoming requirement and where appropriate, assist in its implementation.

7.1.2 Credentialling of providers who use fluoroscopy

According to the Joint Commission, licensed practitioners who provide care and services without direction or supervision within the scope of their license must undergo a process of called credentialling by the organization where they provide care. This helps protect patients from unethical or untrained practitioners by recognizing the competency of a professional. This is a process of obtaining, verifying and assessing the qualifications of a practitioner to provide specific care or services within the organization. This process involves examination of the applicant's education, training, licensure, experience and other appropriate qualifications. Once these have been evaluated, the practitioner may be granted privileges to perform a specific scope and content of patient care services by the organization. A "privilege" is defined as an advantage, right or benefit not available to everyone; the rights and advantages enjoyed by a relatively small group of people, usually as a result of education, training and/or experience [17].

The Accreditation Council for Graduate Medical Education (ACGME) sets and monitors the professional education standards essential in preparing physicians to deliver safe, high-quality medical care in the U.S. [18]. To demonstrate competency in a specific discipline, a practitioner must complete an ACGME-accredited training program and pass an examination in the discipline administered by an independent medical specialty board (e.g., American Board of Radiology, American Board of Surgery, etc.).

Not all graduate medical training programs provide training in the safe use of fluoroscopy. Thus, a practitioner may have used fluoroscopy during his/her residency training and may be technically proficient in its use but have little or no knowledge of how X rays are produced and the hazards they present to the patient, the operator, and other personnel in the room. This can result in the overuse of radiation during a procedure, resulting in unnecessary exposure to both the patient and the practitioner.

A solution is to require training and credentialling of practitioners for the use of fluoroscopy. The FDA advisory discussed above included the following recommendations for operators [6]

- Be trained and understand system operation, including implications for radiation exposure from each mode of operation;
- Be educated so that, on case-by-case basis, assess the risks and benefits for individual patients;
- Counsel patients on symptoms and risks of large radiation exposures and address risks from radiation in the consent form; and
- Be able to justify and limit the use of high dose rate modes of operation.

Some regulatory agencies have mandated training for operators. The State of California Department of Public Health requires practitioners who use or supervise the use of fluoroscopy to obtain a separate license as a Fluoroscopy Supervisor and Operator [19]. Continuing education is required to maintain this license. The City of New York Department of Health regulations require training of all persons operating, or supervising the operation of, fluoroscopy systems (see below) [20].

AAPM Task Group Report No. 124 provides guidelines for establishing a credentialling and privileging program for users of fluoroscopy [21]. This effort will require close coordination with and approval of the organization's Chief Medical Officer (CMO) and the office that oversees the process. The RSO can collaborate with this office to evaluate the provider's credentials and advise the credentialling office on the appropriateness of the request, arrange for training, issue radiation monitoring devices, and ensure appropriate personal protective equipment (i.e., lead or lead equivalent protective aprons and eye wear) is available for the individual.

7.2 Optimizing equipment and processes

7.2.1 Role of the Radiation Safety Officer

As the chief radiological compliance officer of the institution, the RSO oversees the quality assurance program for medical imaging equipment. As such, when regulators inspect the facility the RSO will be held to account for any findings or violations. Therefore, while not directly responsible for performance evaluations, the RSO should audit the program to ensure that they were performed on time and in compliance with regulations, standards, and best practices. The RSO should have the authority to remove from service any equipment that is a radiological safety hazard to patients, staff, or the public. This will ensure the equipment is functioning as designed and will not overexpose patients or staff.

The RSO is also responsible for overseeing the training in radiation safety that is mandated by many regulatory agencies. Training should include

- Awareness of the magnitude of the radiation dose delivered by imaging equipment
- Location of scattered radiation around the patient and in the imaging suite;
- Features of imaging equipment, particularly fluoroscopy units, whose use may reduce patient exposure
- Requirements for monitoring radiation dose to staff and use of personal protective equipment when appropriate
- Policies and procedures relevant to equipment selection and use.

However, this is the minimum expected of the RSO. As an advocate for patient safety, the RSO should proactively seek out ways to optimize processes to reduce patient dose.

7.2.2 Management of patient doses

7.2.2.1 Benchmarking radiation doses

It is well known that there is substantial variation in radiation dose between procedures within an institution and for the sample procedure between healthcare facilities [22]. Efforts to apply ALARA principles to medical imaging and interventional procedures need to appreciate that patient size, region to be image and the clinical indications for the study will affect the radiographic technique(s) and hence, patient dose. Collecting information about radiation doses from potentially high dose procedures will assist the RSO to determine where to prioritize dose reduction efforts. Comparing these results to published data (i.e., benchmarking) will help the RSO to identify best practices and help uncover gaps in knowledge or processes in the institution that can be addressed. These published data are known as diagnostic reference levels (DRLs). For example, in 1999 the European Commission published a guide to member states on the establishment of DRLs [23]. Once established, these levels are "...not to be exceeded for standard procedures when good and normal practice regarding diagnostic and technical performance is applied." This publication also includes example DRLs collected from multiple institutions in 10 member countries.

In the United States, the ACR offers accreditation for a variety of imaging modalities, include CT and mammography. Accreditation ensures the facility is providing the highest level of image quality and safety. For example, as part of the CT accreditation application process, the facility must provide examples of CT protocols for specific procedures with measured and calculated radiation doses [24]. These doses can be used by the facility to benchmark its CT scanners against similar scanners at other sites.

Once DRLs have been established, the RSO can work collaboratively to implement routine collection and reporting of patient doses. This data can be used to develop and implement standard protocols for typical imaging procedures. These protocols should be reviewed routinely to ensure that the institution is taking advantage of the most recently published best practices. If a DRL is consistently exceeded, an investigation should be initiated, and appropriate action taken.

7.2.2.2 Regulatory changes

Changes in regulations may mandate closer supervision of patient radiation doses. For example, the City of New York Department Health and Mental Hygiene completely repealed and re-enacted the radiation control regulations (Article 175 of the New York City Health Code [20]). The changes are numerous and of a broad scope and will significantly increase the administrative and safety oversight burden on the imaging facility. Although many of these changes are focused on occupational exposure to ionizing radiation, several – including requirements for initial and ongoing training of fluoroscopy users – are focused on patient safety.

These regulations do not apply to facilities outside of New York City, but they provide a road map for future regulations in other state jurisdictions. They also provide a list of suggestions for the RSO to consider for the patient radiation dose reduction efforts.

7.2.2.3 Optimization of patient dose

A limited review of the literature suggests that there are steps that can be taken to reduce patient dose, over and above simply ensuring that imaging equipment functions as designed and is operated within standards and regulations.

In a study of radiation dose reduction measures in a busy invasive cardiovascular laboratory [25], investigators achieved a 40% reduction in the mean cumulative skin dose to patients over a three-year period by

- Educating staff about properly adjusting imaging equipment and minimizing duration of beam activation
- Verbally announcing air-kerma values at specific levels with the expectation that further strategies for dose management would be implemented
- Adding air-kerma values to the final report of each procedure
- Investigating relationship between image quality and radiation dose and implementing strategies to maintain acceptable image quality while keeping patient dose to the minimum necessary to achieve the goals of the imaging procedure
- Increased use of copper x-ray beam spectral filters
- Reducing the fluoroscopy frame rate from 15 frames/s to 7.5 frames/s
- Recording and maintain on file radiation dose records by procedure and provider

The U.S. Veterans Administration National Center for Patient Safety (NCPS) (Ann Arbor, MI) funded a study to apply the principles of Healthcare Failure Mode and Effect Analysis (HFMEA), developed by NCPS, to identify systematic gaps associated with potentially high–radiation dose fluoroscopic procedures, to assess the relative importance of different interventions to reduce dose, and to identify areas to improve patient safety [26]. As an example high-radiation dose intervention, they chose to evaluate a pacemaker or implantable cardioverter defibrillator lead extraction procedure. A total of 29 actions were devised of which 5 were determined to be of the highest priority for implementation to reduce patient dose

- Develop a checklist that includes assessment and documentation of clinical risk factors for radiation injury to patients
- Incorporate review of these risk factors into procedural time-outs
- Assign a staff member to verbally notify the operator at medically appropriate times when dose thresholds have been reached. The operator must verbally acknowledge each notification.
- Monitor the skin radiation dose or, if the peak skin dose is not displayed, the reference point air kerma (in milligrays)
- For each type of procedure typically performed, develop an imaging protocol that specifies the machine settings (technique factors); require physicists periodically perform a protocol review, with collection of data, such as radiation outputs for fluoroscopy and image recording.

These are but two examples of efforts by institutions to conduct a detailed analysis of their processes, procedures and equipment function to understand where, why, and how high radiation doses occur and what measures can be implemented to effect reductions. The RSO can bring these and other studies to the attention of both physicians and managers of the interventional cardiology department in their institution.

7.3 Resources for the RSO

There are several resources available to the RSO on the internet. They can be used to educate providers, managers, and medical physicists and focus attention on the need to manage radiation dose to patients. These resources provide guidance and suggestions for implementing change.

7.3.1 Image Gently® campaign

Formed in 2006, Image Gently® is a physician-led initiative begun as a committee within the Society for Pediatric Radiology (SPR). Today, more than 50 medical, dental, and allied professional societies from across the globe have joined as alliance organizations [27]. Like the Image Wisely® campaign discussed below, the goal of this initiative is to change practice by raising awareness of opportunities to reduce radiation dose with a focus on imaging of children. Implementation includes providing information and free educational materials.

7.3.2 Image Wisely® campaign

Image Wisely® is a joint initiative of the American College of Radiology (ACR), Radiological Society of North America (RSNA), American Society of Radiologic Technologists (ASRT) and American Association of Physicists in Medicine (AAPM). Formed to address concerns about the surge of public exposure to ionizing radiation from medical imaging, its objective is to lower the amount of radiation used in medically necessary imaging studies and eliminating unnecessary procedures [28]. The campaign is focused on adult patients. It provides radiation safety information by imaging modality for patients and providers. A free series of online and mobile-compatible education modules are available that include case-based questions that allow the viewer to improve, and then assess, understanding of important safety concepts in medical imaging.

Imaging professionals, referring providers, image facilities, and associations and educational programs are encouraged to sign a pledge to educate themselves on radiation doses from imaging procedures, consulting with professionals prior to ordering studies, optimize dose to ensure only necessary amounts are used to produce images tailored to patient size and the diagnostic task, prevent duplication of exams, and to actively promote these goals among colleagues, staff, members and students.

7.3.3 Bonn Call for Action

In 2012, the IAEA issued the Call for Action at an international conference on radiation protection in medicine in Bonn, Germany [29]. The goal of the conference was to

- Indicate gaps in current approaches to radiation protection in medicine;
- Identify tools for improving radiation protection in medicine;
- Review advances, challenges, and opportunities in this field; and
- Assess the impact of the Call for Action in order to prepare new recommendations.

The Bonn Call for Action Implementation Toolkit is an online platform offering resources for improving radiation protection in medicine that was created as a result of a follow-on conference in 2017. It includes educational resources for referring physicians, radiology and nuclear medicine providers and other professionals, medical physicists, manufacturers, and regulators [30].

Author details

Thomas L. Morgan* and Sandy Konerth
Versant Medical Physics and Radiation Safety, Kalamazoo, MI, USA

*Address all correspondence to: morgantl@aol.com

References

[1] National Council on Radiation Protection and Measurements (NCRP). Ionizing radiation exposure of the population of the United States. NCRP Report 93, Bethesda, MD, 1987.

[2] National Council on Radiation Protection and Measurements (NCRP). Ionizing radiation exposure of the population of the United States. NCRP Report 160, Bethesda, MD, 2009.

[3] National Council on Radiation Protection and Measurements (NCRP). Medical radiation exposure of patients in the United States. NCRP Report 184, Bethesda, MD, 2019.

[4] Fazel R, Krumholtz KM, Wang Y, Ross JS, Chen J, Ting HH, Shah ND, Nasir K, Einstein AJ, Nallamothu BK. Exposure to low-dose ionizing radiation from medical imaging procedures. New Eng J Med 2009;361:849-857. DOI: 10.1056/NEJMoa0901249.

[5] Martin E, Prasarn M, Coyne E, Giordano B, Morgan T, Westessen P-L, Wright J, Rechtine II G. Inpatient radiation exposure in patients with spinal trauma. J Spin Cord Med 2013;36:112-117. DOI: 10.1179/2045772312Y.0000000054.

[6] Food and Drug Administration. Important information for physicians and other health care professionals. Avoidance of serious x-ray-induced skin injuries to patients during fluoroscopically-guided procedures. September 9, 1994 [Internet]. Available from: https://www.fda.gov/downloads/Radiation-EmittingProducts/RadiationEmittingProductsandProcedures/MedicalImaging/MedicalX-Rays/ucm116677.pdf. [Accessed: 2021-02-24]

[7] Brenner DJ, Elliston CD, Hall, EJ, Berdon WE. Estimated risk of radiation-induced fatal cancer from pediatric CT. Amer J Radiol 2001;176:289-296. DOI:10.2214/ajr.176.2.1760289.

[8] Pearce MS, Salotti JA, Little MP, McHugh K, Lee C, Kim PK, Howe NL, Ronckers CM, Rajaraman P, Craft AW, Parker L, Berrington de Gonzalez A. Radiation exposure from CT scans in childhood and subsequent risk of leukemia and brain tumors: a retrospective cohort study. Lancet 2012;380:499-505. DOI:10.1016/S0140-6736(12)60815-0.

[9] Mathews JD, Forsythe AV, Brady Z, Butler MW, Goergen SK, Byrnes GB, Giles GG, Wallace AB, Anderson PR, Guiver TA, McGale P, Cain TM, Dowty JG, Bickerstaffe AC, Darby SC. Cancer risk in 680,000 people exposed to computed tomography scans in childhood or adolescence: data linkage study of 11 million Australians. Brit Med J 2013;346:f2360. DOI: 10.1136/bmj.f2360.

[10] United States Nuclear Regulatory Commission regulation 10 CFR 20.1003. Definitions [Internet]. Available from: https://www.nrc.gov/reading-rm/doc-collections/cfr/part020/part020-1003.html [Accessed: 2021-02-24]

[11] International Council on Radiation Protection (ICRP). Radiological protection and safety in Medicine. ICRP Publication 73. Ann ICRP 1996;26(2). Elsevier Science Inc., Tarrytown, NY.

[12] American Association of Physicists in Medicine (AAPM). The report of Task Group 100 of the AAPM: Application of risk analysis methods to radiation therapy quality management [Internet]. Available from: https://aapm.onlinelibrary.wiley.com/doi/full/10.1118/1.4947547 [Accessed: 2020-12-26]

[13] Centers for Medicare & Medicaid Services. Appropriate use criteria program [Internet]. Available from: https://www.cms.gov/Medicare/Quality-Initiatives-Patient-Assessment-Instruments/Appropriate-Use-Criteria-Program [Accessed: 2021-02-24]

[14] American College of Radiology. ACR Appropriateness Criteria [Internet]. Available from: https://www.acr.org/Clinical-Resources/ACR-Appropriateness-Criteria [Accessed: 2021-02-24]

[15] American Society of Nuclear Cardiology. Appropriate use criteria [Internet]. Available from: https://www.asnc.org/guidelinesandstandards [Accessed: 2021-02-24]

[16] Society of Nuclear Medicine and Molecular Imaging. Appropriate use criteria [Internet]. Available from: https://www.snmmi.org/ClinicalPractice/content.aspx?ItemNumber=15666&navItemNumber=10791 [Accessed: 2021-02-24]

[17] Ambulatory Care Program: The who, what, when, and where's of credentialling and privileging [Internet]. Available from: https://www.jointcommission.org/-/media/deprecated-unorganized/imported-assets/tjc/system-folders/blogs/ahc_who_what_when_and_where_credentialing_bookletpdf.pdf?db=web&hash=CD838EB80D69FE2FA517285B4F3A0537 [Accessed: 2021-02-24]

[18] Accreditation Council for Graduate Medical Education. About Us [Internet]. Available from: https://www.acgme.org/About-Us/Overview [Accessed: 2021-02-24]

[19] Title 17 California Code of Regulations Section 30464. Requirements for radiography permits [Internet]. Available from: https://govt.westlaw.com/calregs/Document/I8C393B90391E11E3A497C9CEC9EBAB68?viewType=FullText&originationContext=documenttoc&transitionType=CategoryPageItem&contextData=(sc.Default) [Accessed: 2021-02-24]

[20] New York City Health Code Section 175.53. Fluoroscopic equipment [Internet]. Available from: https://www1.nyc.gov/assets/doh/downloads/pdf/about/healthcode/health-code-article175.pdf [Accessed: 2021-02-24]

[21] American Association of Physicists in Medicine. A guide for establishing a credentialling and privileging program for users of fluoroscopic equipment in healthcare organizations [Internet]. Available from: https://www.aapm.org/pubs/reports/RPT_124.pdf [Accessed: 2021-02-24]

[22] International Atomic Energy Agency. Radiation Protection of Patients: Justification and optimization [Internet]. Available from: https://www.iaea.org/resources/rpop/resources/international-safety-standards/justification-and-optimization#4 [Accessed: 2021-02-24]

[23] European Commission. Radiation Protection 109: Guidance on diagnostic reference levels (DRLs) for medical exposures [Internet]. Available from: https://ec.europa.eu/energy/sites/ener/files/documents/109_en.pdf [Accessed 2021-02-24]

[24] American College of Radiology. Accreditation information for CT [Internet]. Available from: https://www.acraccreditation.org/Modalities/CT [Accessed: 2021-02-24]

[25] Fetterly KA, Matthew V, Lennon R, Bell MR, Holmes Jr DR, Rihal CS. Radiation dose reduction in the invasive cardiovascular laboratory: Implementing a culture and philosophy of radiation Safety. JACC: Cardiovas Interven 2012;5:866-873. DOI: 10.1016/j.jcin.2012.05.0

[26] Justinvil GN, Leidholdt Jr EM, Balter S, Graves, LL, Loring BA, Brenner AC, Boyle NG, Srinivasa RN, Moran JM. Preventing harm from fluoroscopically guided interventional procedures with a risk-based analysis approach. J Am Coll Radiol 2019;16:1144-1152. DOI: 10.1016/j.jacr.2019.02.047

[27] Image Gently [Internet]. Available from: https://www.imagegently.org/ [Accessed: 2021-02-24]

[28] Image Wisely [Internet]. Available from: https://www.imagewisely.org/ [Accessed: 2021-02-24]

[29] Bonn Call for Action [Internet]. Available from: https://www.iaea.org/resources/rpop/resources/bonn-call-for-action-platform [Accessed: 2021-02-24]

[30] Bonn Call for Action implementation toolkit [Internet]. Available from: https://gnssn.iaea.org/main/bonn-toolkit/SitePages/Home.aspx [Accessed: 2021-02-24]

Chapter 6

Safety and Potential Risks with Fecal Microbiota Transplantation

Pratyusha Gaonkar

Abstract

The therapeutic potential of Fecal Microbiota Transplantation (FMT) is greatly proved worldwide in the recent years. The use of FMT is now an accepted treatment modality and effective standard of care for some patients owing to its success in treating recurrent *Clostridium Difficile* Infection (rCDI). However, it is still evolving and longer term follow-up data regarding safety are required. Post-FMT serious adverse events (SAEs) have been varied between studies, however have included significant morbidity necessitating hospital admission and mortality in the follow-up period. The follow-up of FMT recipients should be long enough to completely establish efficacy/adverse events. Furthermore, it is recommended that FMT should be offered with caution to immunosuppressed patients, in whom FMT appears efficacious without significant additional adverse effects. In the wake of COVID-19 situation, stringent policies in screening the FMT donors have to be put forth to ensure patient safety. There is a need for high-quality, large, prospective, randomized controlled trials and long-term follow-up investigating screened donors and recipients to evaluate the long term safety and the risk–benefit profile of this promising therapy.

Keywords: safety, risks, fecal, microbiota, adverse events, COVID-19

1. Introduction

Owing to the success of Fecal Microbiota Transplantation (FMT) in treating various diseases, there's a growing demand for standardizing the preparation of fecal material, using accepted standards for the delivery, ensuring safety for the recipient, and monitoring long-term outcomes [1]. The most robust clinical evidence is driven by studies of FMT as a treatment for refractory or recurrent *Clostridium difficile* infection (CDI). Despite the progress in studying the FMT therapy in CDI, there are no prospective studies assessing the safety or efficacy of FMT in IBD. However, critics still have significant concerns regarding the acceptability of FMT, the ethical issues associated with risk and studying FMT in patients with severe disease [2]. Despite the enthusiasm regarding FMT research, the pertinent questions remain, apart from those addressing potential therapeutic indications. These comprise whether the TM could be whole flora extract or cultured TM, methods of administration, implantation success, and immunologic responses, as well as the long-term safety implications of altering the microbiota composition [3]. In the first clinical trial that assessed this treatment modality, FMT proved so superior to standard antibiotics that the study's data and safety monitoring board stopped enrollment early, concluding that it was unethical to hold back the treatment from the members of the control group. However, it is crucial to understand that diseases that have been linked to the microbiome may surface years post the procedure. As such, there remains a requirement for more investigation of the safety profile of FMT in the extreme long term [4].

2. Safety concerns and the significance of donor screening protocol

FMT as a treatment modality is considered unique owing to the difficulty of its characterization and the simplicity of its production, and each of these characteristics raises special safety concerns. First, the complexity of the communities of microbes in stool and the variability across samples makes it challenging to guarantee the contents from one batch to another. Per se, ongoing monitoring with regards to the presence of possible pathogens is vital for maintaining a safe product and should either be considered part of the approved manufacturing process or a condition imposed on manufacturers. Second, even though there is little scope that patients will manufacture traditional small molecule therapies in their lavatories, processing stool for transplantation at a basic level needs very little training or equipment. Patient online forums comprise lengthy thorough instructions coupled with discussions regarding best practices for mixing stool in a low-cost blender and administering it through enema. There is a considerable risk of pathogen transmission from improperly screened and handled tool due to unsupervised, do-it-yourself procedures. Few healthy subjects would be considered eligible for stool donation for fecal transplantation. Only six per cent of prospective donors to OpenBiome clear the full screening process. This includes a thorough 109-item clinical evaluation administered by a nurse or physician, and 30 stool and blood screens. It is wise to be very cautious about screening for diseases that are potentially transmitted by the microbiome. For instance, investigators have notably linked the microbiome to diverse parameters such as obesity, metabolic syndrome, and behavior. Likewise, it is just as crucial to accumulate longitudinal safety data to identify any conditions that may be transmitted via stool of which we are unaware. Thus, taking into account the known and unknown risks that come with improper donor screening and inadequate patient follow-up, the ease with which patients may prepare and administer fecal transplants themselves without medical supervision, any regulatory outcome that results in restricted access by either limiting supply or significantly increasing the cost of therapy should be adopted very cautiously [4]. Hence, donor screening protocol is a crucial step. Preferred stool donors are healthy individuals without pre-existing disease or risk factors for disease. These individuals are recruited by stool banks and undergo a detailed screening process that includes a questionnaire to exclude those with disease, exposure to transmissible diseases, or behavioral risk factors for transmissible diseases. Disease exclusions comprise, but are not limited to, blood- or stool-borne infections, gastrointestinal disorders, malignancy, atopy, metabolic syndrome and autoimmune diseases. Individuals who have recently taken antibiotics or have traveled to areas with a high risk of traveler's diarrhea are excluded [5].

3. The gaps in understanding FMT safety risk

Many researchers state that FMT is "safe" based on a multitude of uncontrolled trials without a placebo control. Closer examination of adverse event (AE) reporting, however, recommends a need for caution on several grounds. Some of the factors that could be responsible for these gaps are potential under-reporting of adverse events and the uncontrolled design of FMT trials [6]. In the largest FMT trial so far, 219 subjects (mean age, 73 years) were randomized to fresh or frozen FMT via enema. Six deaths (5.6%) occurred in the frozen FMT arm, and 11 deaths (11.7%) occurred in the fresh FMT arm; none were attributed by the investigators to FMT [7]. Although the CDI morbidity and mortality rates have been reported to be as high as 15%, it is difficult to understand which AEs may be treatment-related without the benefit of a placebo-controlled arm [6]. A few FMT proponents have debated that some patient subgroups, such as immunocompromised hosts, often do not qualify for placebo-controlled trials and need open access to FMT [8]. Still, implicit in this statement is the implication that FMT has been demonstrated to be efficacious and safe in this patient population when there are no controlled trials to support such assumptions. Furthermore, comparison of AE rates between 2 FMT products is useful [6]. In a randomized, double-blind, placebo-controlled phase 2B trial of a stool-derived microbiome drug product, RBX2660, 64% of recurrent CDI patients reported an AE; the distribution of these AEs was comparable by treatment arm (2 doses of placebo vs. 2 doses RBX2660 vs. 1 dose RBX2660/placebo) [9]. On the other hand, a stool bank (OpenBiome, Cambridge, MA, USA) reported 42 AEs in 2050 subjects who underwent FMT, for an event rate of 2%. Besides, none of the AEs was judged to be "definitely related to FMT". Attributing the dramatic differences in event rates to major differences in the products themselves is challenging, as both are stool-derived. The main differences seem to be the methodologies used in collection of AEs and reporting. In the randomized placebo-controlled phase 2b trial of RBX2660, AEs were systematically collected on a prospective basis and investigators were mandated to allocate causality [6]. On the contrary, OpenBiome asks clinicians to retrospectively report, and the stool bank portrays the association of the product to AEs rather than the clinicians [6, 10]. This kind of methodology is disposed to bias. There is a chance of retrospective reporting missing the links between infections and FMT if the patient is assessed by a different health care provider who does not recognize the temporal relationship [6]. Serial FMT Interventions with invasive procedures is another matter to worry about. A trial reported 90% efficacy in 20 subjects managed with FMT, although on delving into the article, it was found that the first-dose efficacy was only 65% [11]. In order to reach 90% efficacy, multiple infusions (2–4 per patient) were given. Repeat infusions through invasive techniques such as colonoscopy, should also be weighed in the risk/benefit analysis of any procedure, and first dose efficacy rates need to be reported with clarity [6].

4. Safety of FMT in *C. difficile* infections

Arguably the best example of harnessing the gut microbiota to manage a disease is the use of F) for the treatment of CDI, where the most convincing safety and efficacy data for use of FMT has shifted the treatment paradigm and revolutionized its management [12]. Most patients with CDI are aged and often with present with co-morbidities, but many other recipients of FMT are likely to be much younger. For such patients, the long-term consequences of gut microbiome manipulation have yet to be understood. There are, for instance, anecdotal reports of numerous changes that have occurred post FMT [13]. These include reversal of immune thrombocytopenic purpura and neurological symptom reversal in three patients with multiple sclerosis [14, 15]. In two patients, the resistant coliforms present before FMT were supplanted by ciprofloxacin-sensitive coliforms after FMT. FMT for refractory CDI lead to an apparent improvement in the related urinary organisms exhibiting 'significantly decreased drug resistance.' This was further supported by two case reports using FMT to decolonize patients with multi-drug-resistant carbapenemase-producing strains of *Klebsiella pneumoniae*. Other researchers have observed improvement in pre-existing allergic sinusitis and arthritis. In a case series of patients with Crohn's disease treated with FMT, eight out of 11 patients noted relief of concomitant 'skin lesions', a phenomenon also observed in another group using FMT to treat ulcerative colitis where three cases demonstrated improvement in 'skin problems' as well as decreased insulin requirements in a diabetic patient. Furthermore, a case report has been published linking FMT to the development of obesity [13]. FMT for recurrent *C. difficile* possesses a good short-term safety record. Very few adverse effects are directly attributed to the procedure. Most reported adverse events have been self-limiting gastrointestinal symptoms comprising abdominal cramps, diarrhea and constipation, which resolved within one week. At least two deaths from aspiration pneumonia related to sedation administered at the time of FMT have been reported. At least one death from transmission of a multidrug resistant *Escherichia coli* organism has been reported, however the donor in this case had not been tested for this organism. However, these deaths are relatively less compared to the large number of FMTs performed [5]. A long-term follow-up study by Brandt et al., patients who had colonoscopic FMT for RCDI≥3 months before the study were asked to completed a 36-item questionnaire that solicited pre-FMT, post-FMT and donor data. Out of 77, 4 patients reported a new medical condition after FMT including peripheral neuropathy, Sjogren's disease, idiopathic thrombocytopenic purpura and rheumatoid arthritis. A total of 7 of the 77 patients died at the time of the study. The causes of death were metastatic colon cancer (present before FMT), metastatic ovarian cancer, pneumonia (secondary to non-enteric organism), myocardial infarction, stroke, sepsis in a patient with longstanding CD 5 months after FMT, and one patient deceased while on hospice care from unknown cause. None of these causes seemed to be attributable to FMT [16, 17].

5. Safety of FMT in ulcerative colitis (UC)

UC, a major subtype of IBD, perhaps denotes one of the most robust potential indications for FMT after RCDI [18]. Rossen et al. evaluated the efficacy and safety of FMT in 37 patients with UC in a double-blind randomized trial, and noted mild adverse events in the majority of patients (64%), including transient borborygmus (49%), increased stool frequency (34%), vomiting in 2 patients and transient fever in 2 patients. Most adverse events resolved spontaneously within 2 days. There were no infectious complications observed. Four SAEs happened, but were not related to FMT itself. It has been noted that some patients develop self-limited fever and temporary elevation of CRP and IL-6 following FMT, but were considered non-significant, as patients did not show deterioration [16]. Fang et al. concluded that single fresh FMT is an effective and safe strategy to induce long-term remission in patients with active UC and could be expected to be an alternative induction therapy for recurrent UC, even primary UC. None of the patients suffered from other chronic diseases such as immune system diseases, non-alcoholic fatty liver disease and all patients demonstrated good tolerance to FMT treatment [18].

6. Safety of FMT in inflammatory bowel disease (IBD)

Owing to its success in treating rCDI, the use of FMT became rapidly accepted [1]. It appears that most patients with IBD managed with FMT for RCDI tolerate the procedure well; nevertheless, there appears to be a potential risk of precipitating a flare. Whether this flare is related to FMT or as part of the natural course of IBD is ambiguous [16]. In a retrospective case series by Kelly et al., a few patients with IBD were reported to present with 'IBD flare' post FMT (14%). It is worth nothing that patients with IBD did not experience a higher incidence of SAEs (11%) or adverse events (14%) compared with patient immunocompromised due to other conditions (18% SAEs, 16% AEs, $p \leq 0.3224$) [19]. The definite mechanism of IBD flare post FMT is still ambiguous, although Quera et al. suggested that transient bacteremia may lead to an altered intestinal permeability, resulting in a flare [20]. In their open-label, single-center prospective trial, Goyal et al., concluded that a single FMT is relatively safe and can result in a short-term response in young patients with active IBD. Samples from responders had significantly increased Fusobacterium prior to FMT and showed more significant microbiome changes compared with non-responders after FMT [21]. Further research is needed to discern whether the abundance of Fusobacterium, an organism associated with numerous adverse health outcomes, has prognostic value in the setting of FMT for IBD [22].

7. Safety of FMT in immunocompromised patients

The safety of using live microorganisms in a treatment modality such as FMT remains unclear in certain patient groups—particularly, in severely immunosuppressed patients [23]. Few experts are concerned that there may be a greater risk for infection post FMT in patients with immunocompromised status. Kelly et al. examined FMT in 80 immunocompromised patients of CDI and observed that there were no infection events related to FMT while high cure rates of 78% following a single FMT were noted [20]. Among the different FMT delivery methods used, there were no observed differences in the proportion of adverse events [7, 24, 25]. Nevertheless, long-term immunologic effects of FMT is another matter of concern, but very little relevant data is available [20]. Numerous case reports have indicated that there might be some undetermined association between FMT and certain conditions, including peripheral neuropathy, idiopathic thrombocytopenic purpura, Sjogren's syndrome, and rheumatoid arthritis [17]. Presently, the definite periodicity and duration of follow-up post FMT for monitoring of long-term adverse events are not established. The European consensus proposed that the follow-up period post FMT in CDI patients should be minimum 8 weeks, and the contents of follow-up must comprise clinical and analytical information [26].

8. Adverse events reported in past clinical literature

Most clinical trials and systematic reviews demonstrated that some minor adverse events, like abdominal discomfort, diarrhea, constipation, and low-grade fever, were transiently observed post FMT, whereas uncommon severe side effects were often related to the possible complications of endoscopy and sedation [20, 27–29]. According to the past clinical literature, the two most common side effects of FMT observed are bloating and loose stools for the first 24 hours. These usually resolve soon thereafter and most patients usually have formed stool by 1–2 weeks. The clinicians do not recommend stool testing for resolution in those with formed stool, but is considered if 3 or more diarrhea stools per day occur post few weeks. It is crucial to note that the polymerase chain reaction test for *C. difficile* toxin may remain positive for 30 days after a successful treatment, which is another reason not to test asymptomatic patients who underwent FMT. An unclear presentation is abdominal cramping and intermittent frequent bowel movements occurring in a patient who might be a carrier of *C. difficile* and who is a FMT recipient. These patients are most likely to have post-infectious IBS. Hence, the clinician should ideally be able to differentiate between post-infectious IBS and rCDI in order to avoid unnecessarily repetition of FMT [1]. In a systematic review by Marcella et al., FMT-related adverse events were summarized. (**Table 1**) Largely, 85 unique types of AEs were reported in 24% of FMT procedures (1347/5688) during or after FMT, including 6% (246/4241) of patients with SAEs [30].

Although FMT may seem "natural" and safe, possibly even "frugal," clinicians are concerned about the long-term effects that donors' intestinal microbes may have on patients receiving FMT [31]. For instance, the gut microbiota has been shown to be a possible transferrable agent of risk or phenotype in multiple disorders, including obesity, cardiovascular disease, and autoimmune disorders, such as type 1 diabetes [32, 33]. Furthermore, the gut microbiota has been found to interact with the central nervous system and to affect brain chemistry and behaviors [34]. Theoretically, FMT could bring about the transmission of anxiety and depression,

Adverse Events	% of Patients Affected
Diarrhea	10.00%
Abdominal discomfort, Cramping, Pain	7.35%
Nausea, Vomiting	3.31%
Excessive flatulence,	3.23%
Constipation	1.90%
Fever	1.71%
Fatigue, Malaise	1.32%
Fecal urgency	0.76%
Proctalgia	0.46%
Endoscopy-related respiratory difficulties	0.39%
Disease relapse	0.37%
Regurgitation Belching,	0.33%
Disease exacerbation	0.28%
Bloody Stool	0.21%
Sore throat, Rash, Skin erythema, Pruritus	0.14%
Anorectal discomfort, Headache	0.12%
Aspiration pneumonia, CMV infection, Rectal bleeding, Chills	0.11%
Bacteremia, Death	0.09%
Mucoid stool, Transient borborygmus	0.07%
Diverticulitis	0.05%
Peripheral Neuropathy, Norovirus gastroenteritis, Rhinorrhea, Herpes zoster, Decreased appetite, Dizziness, *C. perfringens* Infection	0.03%
Sjogren's disease, ITP, Rheumatoid arthritis, Minor mucosal tear during colonoscopy, Hematemesis, Chest distress, Testicular pain, Myasthenia gravis, Hot flashes, Allergic bronchitis, Dehydration, Rectal prolapse, Appendicitis, URTI, Pancreatitis, Stuffy nose, Depression, Anorexia, Soling of transplant, Vertigo	0.02%

Table 1.
FMT related adverse events [30].

autism, or neurological conditions, such as Parkinson's disease. However, most of these effects have only been observed in preclinical studies [32].

9. The different AEs report in randomized controlled trials (RCTs) and non-controlled studies

In a systematic review by Marcella et al., twenty studies of RCTs included 558 patients: 222 with IBS, 138 with UC, 70 with CDI and few patients with cirrhosis, constipation, obesity, autism spectrum disorder and hepatic encephalopathy. While in non-controlled studies, the most common indication was CDI followed by IBD. When compared to RCTs, non-controlled studies demonstrated a lower trend of FMT-related AEs rate. Nevertheless, all FMT-related SAEs were reported in non-controlled studies. This result should not be considered as a premise as patients with severe cases or immunocompromised were essentially excluded from RCT. Therefore, RCT results should not be referred to as the representative as a whole.

10. AEs in populations with different delivery route

The incidence of FMT-related AEs by route of delivery comprised colonic transendoscopic enteral tubing (TET) (6%), colonoscopy (15%), enema (26%), capsule (29%), midgut tube (29%) and gastroscopy (32%). Upon analysis, the incidence of FMT-related AEs was more common in patients who had FMT via the upper GI routes than lower GI routes (28.8% vs. 17.5%). This result is in conjunction with the incidence of FMT-related SAEs in upper and lower GI route (1.4% vs. 0.9%). Additionally, the SAEs that occurred in FMT recipients via gastroscopy and mid-gut tube were all delivery-related SAEs. This confers to a belief that patients likely experienced SAEs caused by invasive endoscope procedures rather than the microbiota-related SAEs for upper GI routes (except for capsule). On the contrary, for lower GI routes and capsule, a plethora of SAEs were microbiota-related. Kunde et al. outlined the tolerability of FMT in children with UC and intolerance with immediate leaking of enemas happened in one patient. Colonic TET was in recent times used as the delivery of washed microbiota for the elderly, adults and children to ensure the whole-colon administration of microbiota and to meet the patient's needs that required multiple FMTs [30]. AEs such as nausea (1%), pharynx discomfort (5%) and rhinorrhea (1%); and procedure-related: mild pharynx bleeding (1%), epistaxis (5%) and unplanned extubation (2%) were reported in a study comprising patients who underwent mid-gut TET [35]. Ekekezie et al. published a survey regarding do-it-yourself (DIY) FMT that consisted of 84 respondents [36]. The survey demonstrated that DIY FMT was most commonly used in IBD (35%) and IBS (29%) patients. AEs, such as abdominal pain, flatulence and bloating, changes in mood, fever, infection and hospitalization were reported in 12% of the participants. Self-administration of home FMT via enema was observed in two articles, which allowed eight patients to complete 11 courses of FMT in total. About 87.5% (7/8) of patients benefited from this. Three patients developed AEs, two patients had urinary tract infection post-FMT deemed to be not related to the FMT and one patient experienced severe bloody diarrhea, weakness, abdominal pain and weight loss several weeks post-FMT, which was due to CMV infection [30]. CMV is observed in up to one-third of IBD patients with the glucocorticoid-refractory disease [37]. Moreover, CMV may arise inadvertently from an unconventional method of home or self FMT preparation. Hence, there is a need for increased awareness around DIY-FMT and research around this phenomenon, which may leverage public health [30].

11. Informed consent

Informed consent usually presupposes three elements such as capacity to consent, voluntariness, and information [38]. It is not capacity to consent but inadequate information that may pose problems with regards to FMT [32]. In recurrent and refractory CDI cases, FMT could be considered in the "transition zone" between experimental research and standard of care [32, 39]. Even though innovative interventions are generally regulated less strictly than new drugs or biological products, their "experimental" nature does imply special ethical requirements for informed consent [32]. Despite the fact that there are no formal standards for the content of informed consent for "transition zone" interventions, it is usually accepted that such discussions should include the following components: the innovative nature of the procedure, the provider's experience with the procedure, the risk–benefit profile including unknown risks, the (lack of) evidence, and alternatives to the innovative intervention [32, 40].

12. Washed microbiota transplantation

The FMT procedure using washing process was coined as washed microbiota transplantation (WMT). FMT on the basis of washed microbiota preparation has been shown to reduce adverse events caused by traditional fecal suspension preparation and significantly improve the efficacy [41]. Population evidence demonstrated the washed microbiota preparation with microfiltration based on an automatic purification system followed by repeated centrifugation plus suspension for three times significantly decreased the adverse events related to FMT [42]. With the goal to improve the safety of FMT, studies regarding improved methodology of fecal microbiota preparation known as WMT continue to accrue in China since 2014. WMT is based on the principle of automatic filtration and washing process and the related delivery [30, 42, 43]. The improved safety of WMT was reinforced by the metagenomics next-generation sequencing and metabolomics analysis that demonstrated more types, amount of viruses, and pro-inflammatory mediators were washed out during the washing process [30].

13. FMT in the COVID-19 pandemic

Owing to the outbreak of COVID19, healthcare facilities have intensively decreased elective activities both to avoid potential transmission of the virus and to shift human and structural resources to the management of COVID-19 [44]. In the wake of COVID-19 situation, stringent policies in screening the FMT donors have to be put to ensure the patient safety [30]. Due to the potential risk of transmission of SARS-CoV-2 via Fecal Microbiota for Transplantation (FMT), FDA has determined that additional precautions are needed for any investigational use of FMT, whether under an Investigational New Drug Application (IND) on file with the FDA or under FDA's enforcement discretion policy. The following recommendation has been made by FDA. It has already notified all IND holders of the need for additional precautions namely:

No clinical use of FMT product manufactured from stool donated on or post December 1, 2019, until further screening and testing procedures and changes to the informed consent process are implemented for such stool donations as defined below:

1. Screening of stool donor, including an evaluation of whether, since December 1, 2019, the donor was diagnosed with laboratory-confirmed SARS-CoV-2 infection, experienced symptoms of COVID-19 not explained by another diagnosis, or was exposed to a suspected or confirmed case of COVID-19.

    ◦ In any occurrences of suspected or confirmed SARS-CoV-2 infection or exposure as described above, exclusion of the donor from further donations is recommended. Also, it is recommended that there should not be any clinical use of any FMT product manufactured from stool donated by the affected donor beginning 4 weeks prior to the suspected or confirmed SARS-CoV-2 infection or exposure should be avoided.

2. Performing test of the stool donation or stool donor for SARS-CoV-2 virus or RNA.

    ◦ Tests may include testing upper respiratory clinical specimens (e.g., nasal swabs) or other clinical specimens (e.g., rectal swabs or stool donations).

    ◦ If SARS-CoV-2 is identified, exclusion of the donor from further donations is recommended. Also, it is recommended that there should not be any clinical use of any FMT product manufactured from stool donated by the affected donor beginning 4 weeks prior to the first positive test.

3. In the context of informed consent process, it is crucial to convey to the FMT recipient that healthy, asymptomatic stool donors may potentially be infected with SARS-CoV-2, explain the testing approach and other strategies used to alleviate the risk of SARS-CoV-2 transmission, and advise the FMT recipient of the limitations of testing and risk mitigation strategies [45].

In their position paper, Ianiro et al., depending on the available clinical evidence, the panel provided guidance on issues relating to the impact of COVID-19 on FMT, including selection of patient, selection and recruitment of donor, FMT procedures, patient follow-up and further research activities. Few feasible security measures have been proposed in this article so as to assure a safe cohabitation with COVID-19 in the near future. Following are the recommendations for every step of the FMT procedure to mitigate the potential risk of SARS-CoV-2 transmission:

Outpatient assessment:

Remote assessment (teleconsultation) is recommended.

If remote assessment not possible: Checkpoint at entrance (body temperature; patients must wear surgical mask; hand wash; no company admitted) is recommended.

COVID-19 screening (exposure and medical history, symptoms, laboratory analyses) is recommended.

If clinical suspect of COVID-19, nasopharyngeal swab must be carried out.

Inpatient assessment:

Exclusion of COVID-19 via tests. (nasopharyngeal swab, laboratory exams, if fever or respiratory distress conduct chest CT scan).

Isolation is recommended. (contact precautions and droplets in air).

If patient is COVID-19 positive:

- Dedicated COVID-19 wards and dedicated healthcare professionals recommended.

- Dedicated radiology and invasive procedures recommended.
- Assess the risk/benefit profile of FMT procedure.

Donor screening:

Remote evaluation (The screening could be done through teleconsultation).

Screening for COVID-19 (Details about exposure to confirmed cases, medical history, symptoms, if any).

Laboratory examinations are recommended (standard blood and stool tests plus nasopharyngeal swab and serology for SARS-CoV-2).

Donors who test positive must be excluded from donation and previously donated stool, up to 4 weeks before the occurrence of symptoms/COVID-19 diagnosis, should be discarded as initial clinical evidence proposes that SARS-CoV-2 is detected in stools up to 4 weeks post infection.

Sample donation:

A dedicated toilet at the stool bank should be reserved for collection of stool, and high-touch surface areas should be cleaned post each donation.

Repeat standard and COVID-19 screening interview is recommended for donors.

Checkpoint at the entrance (body temperature, subjects must wear surgical mask, hand wash, company forbidden) is recommended.

Direct stool testing for SARS-CoV-2 and/or common pathogens and quarantine approach as potential alternative is recommended.

Sample handling:

Stool sample transferred to laboratory by dedicated healthcare workers is recommended.

Retention of stool samples for 'look-back' testing is suggested.

Stool processing that conforms to local standard operating procedures and biosafety protocols; at minimum, biosafety level 2 is recommended.

FMT using endoscopic procedure:

- Patients undergoing outpatient elective endoscopic FMT should have temperature checked and be questioned about possible symptoms.
- Dedicated healthcare professionals for COVID-19 is recommended.
- Staff present in the endoscopic room must be protected for aerosol generating procedures.
- Patients need to wear surgical mask.
- Outpatient discharged post brief observation, medical and nurse staff report follow-up instructions to caregivers via teleconsultation.

Follow-up:

Follow-up visits should preferably take place via teleconsultation, outpatient visits should be limited to cases where in-presence assessment is mandatory [44].

14. Recommendations for future clinical trials

The safety of any investigational product is best understood with respect to a placebo-controlled trial with appropriate sample size with an adequate follow-up period. A national FMT registry, supported by a grant to the American Gastroenterology Association from the National Institutes of Health, has been initiated to address the limited knowledge of the long-term risks of FMT [6]. This registry aims to collect the efficacy and safety data on 4000 patients who undergo FMT for up to 10 years to understand the long-term risks and benefits of FMT [30]. However, the study results will not be available for many years to come. The important reason for caution regarding potential long-term consequences of FMT is the ever-increasing list of diseases related to the microbiome [6, 46]. Clinicians should be aware of data limitations when counseling patients concerning any investigational therapy. The following recommendations could be made for future FMT based trials and for reporting of data to improve the fundamental understanding of FMT safety and efficacy:

Exclusive employment of toxin testing to ensure selection of patients with true recurrent CDI.

- Enrolment of subjects with acute-onset CDI.
- Consideration of key exclusion criteria such as long-term suppressive antibiotics for CDI.
- Reporting of the number of treatments required to achieve clinical resolution, as repeated FMT treatments carry procedural risks, depending on route of administration.
- Statistical interpretation should take into account loss to follow-up and other AEs that lead to treatment discontinuation, which are considered treatment failures in most clinical trials.
- Large double-blind, placebo-controlled trials are important for adequate evaluation of the efficacy and safety of any investigational intervention, including FMT. On the other hand, future comparator trials with vancomycin pulse-taper regimens should be considered to fully evaluate if FMT offers additional advantages over other recommended therapeutic approaches [6].

15. Concluding remarks

Over the last decade, much progress has been made studying FMT for the management of CDI, and there are multiple ongoing studies also assessing it as a therapy for other conditions. Nonetheless, there is still much to learn regarding the gut microbiome and its role in disease physiology and treatment. Both physicians and patients will benefit from a better understanding of the risks of FMT and delineated protocols to assess adverse events, complications, and follow-up. There is a need for high-quality, large, prospective, randomized controlled trials and long-term follow-up investigating screened donors and recipients to evaluate the long term safety and the risk–benefit profile of this promising therapy [47]. Furthermore, immunocompromised patients represent a special patient population, and designing a randomized controlled trial that addresses the safety and efficacy of FMT among these individuals will definitely be a welcoming step forward [48]. Mandatory stringent screening guidelines for stool donors are the need of the hour, even though screening cannot prevent unanticipated emerging infections [6]. The COVID-19 pandemic is challenging the healthcare systems globally, and it is reasonable to assume that it will be present also in the near future, compelling us to adjust the overall clinical-procedural standards. Lastly, the development of investigational microbiome therapeutics with defined microbial consortia will provide greater confidence in drug purity, identity, and potency, in addition to risk mitigation for improved patient safety [6, 44].

Acknowledgements

None declared.

Conflict of interest

There are no conflicts of interest.

Notes/thanks/other declarations

There are no declarations.

Acronyms and abbreviations

FMT	fecal microbiota transplantation
rCDI	*clostridium difficile* infection
UC	ulcerative colitis
IBD	inflammatory bowel disease
WMT	washed microbiota transplantation
SAEs	serious adverse events
RCTs	randomized controlled trials
SARS-CoV-2	severe acute respiratory syndrome coronavirus 2
TET	transendoscopic enteral tubing

Author details

Pratyusha Gaonkar
Medical Advisor at Lupin Ltd., Mumbai, India

*Address all correspondence to: pratyushagaonkar1@gmail.com

References

[1] Kim KO, Gluck M. Fecal microbiota transplantation: an update on clinical practice. Clinical Endoscopy. 2019 Mar;52(2):137.

[2] Kahn SA, Vachon A, Rodriquez D, Goeppinger SR, Surma B, Marks J, Rubin DT. Patient perceptions of fecal microbiota transplantation for ulcerative colitis. Inflammatory bowel diseases. 2013 Jun 1;19(7):1506-1513.

[3] Borody TJ, Paramsothy S, Agrawal G. Fecal microbiota transplantation: indications, methods, evidence, and future directions. Current gastroenterology reports. 2013 Aug 1;15(8):337.

[4] Sachs RE, Edelstein CA. Ensuring the safe and effective FDA regulation of fecal microbiota transplantation. Journal of Law and the Biosciences. 2015 Jul 13;2(2):396-415.

[5] Soo WT, Bryant RV, Costello SP. Faecal microbiota transplantation: indications, evidence and safety. Australian Prescriber. 2020 Apr;43(2):36.

[6] Wilcox MH, McGovern BH, Hecht GA. The Efficacy and Safety of Fecal Microbiota Transplant for Recurrent Clostridium difficile infection: Current Understanding and Gap Analysis. InOpen Forum Infectious Diseases 2020 May (Vol. 7, No. 5, p. ofaa114). US: Oxford University Press.

[7] Lee CH, Steiner T, Petrof EO, et al. Frozen vs fresh fecal microbiota transplantation and clinical resolution of diarrhea in patients with recurrent Clostridium difficile infection: a randomized clinical trial. JAMA 2016; 315:142-149.

[8] Kelly CR, Fischer M, Grinspan A, et al. Patients eligible for trials of microbebased therapeutics do not represent the population with recurrent Clostridioides difficile infection. Clin Gastroenterol Hepatol. In press.

[9] Dubberke ER, Lee CH, Orenstein R, Khanna S, Hecht G, Gerding DN. Results from a randomized, placebo-controlled clinical trial of a RBX2660—a microbiota-based drug for the prevention of recurrent Clostridium difficile infection. Clinical Infectious Diseases. 2018 Sep 28;67(8):1198-1204.

[10] Glover SC, Burstiner S, Jones D, Teymoorian A, Naga Y, Silver J, Pallav K. E. coliSepsis Following FMT in an IgA Deficient IBD Subject: 2099. American Journal of Gastroenterology. 2019 Oct 1;114(2019 ACG Annual Meeting Abstracts):S1170.

[11] Cammarota G, Masucci L, Ianiro G, Bibbò S, Dinoi G, Costamagna G, Sanguinetti M, Gasbarrini A. Randomised clinical trial: faecal microbiota transplantation by colonoscopy vs. vancomycin for the treatment of recurrent Clostridium difficile infection. Alimentary pharmacology & therapeutics. 2015 May;41(9):835-843.

[12] Krajicek E, Fischer M, Allegretti JR, Kelly CR. Nuts and bolts of fecal microbiota transplantation. Clinical Gastroenterology and Hepatology. 2019 Jan 1;17(2):345-352.

[13] Baxter M, Colville A. Adverse events in faecal microbiota transplant: a review of the literature. Journal of Hospital Infection. 2016 Feb 1;92(2):117-127.

[14] Borody T, Campbell J, Torres M, Nowak A, Leis S. Reversal of idiopathic thrombocytopenic purpura [ITP] with fecal microbiota transplantation [FMT]. Am J Gastroenterol 2011;106:S352

[15] Borody T, Leis S, Campbell J, Torres M, Nowak A. Fecal microbiota

transplantation (FMT) in multiple sclerosis (MS). Am J Gastroenterol 2011;106:S352.

[16] Sbahi H, Di Palma JA. Faecal microbiota transplantation: applications and limitations in treating gastrointestinal disorders. BMJ open gastroenterology. 2016 May 1;3(1).

[17] Brandt LJ, Aroniadis OC, Mellow M, Kanatzar A, Kelly C, Park T, Stollman N, Rohlke F, Surawicz C. Long-Term Follow-Up of Colonoscopic Fecal Microbiota Transplant for RecurrentClostridium difficileInfection. American Journal of Gastroenterology. 2012 Jul 1;107(7):1079-1087.

[18] Fang H, Fu L, Li X, Wang J, Xiong K, Su Y, Zhang L. Long-term efficacy and safety of single fecal microbiota transplantation for recurrent active ulcerative colitis. medRxiv. 2020 Jan 1.

[19] Kelly CR, Ihunnah C, Fischer M, Khoruts A, Surawicz C, Afzali A, Aroniadis O, Barto A, Borody T, Giovanelli A, Gordon S. Fecal microbiota transplant for treatment of Clostridium difficile infection in immunocompromised patients. The American journal of gastroenterology. 2014 Jul;109(7):1065.

[20] Wang JW, Kuo CH, Kuo FC, Wang YK, Hsu WH, Yu FJ, Hu HM, Hsu PI, Wang JY, Wu DC. Fecal microbiota transplantation: review and update. Journal of the Formosan Medical Association. 2019 Mar 1;118:S23–S31.

[21] Goyal A, Yeh A, Bush BR, Firek BA, Siebold LM, Rogers MB, Kufen AD, Morowitz MJ. Safety, clinical response, and microbiome findings following fecal microbiota transplant in children with inflammatory bowel disease. Inflammatory bowel diseases. 2018 Jan 18;24(2):410-421.

[22] Han YW. Fusobacterium nucleatum: a commensal-turned pathogen. Current opinion in microbiology. 2015 Feb 1;23:141-147.

[23] Allegretti JR, Mullish BH, Kelly C, Fischer M. The evolution of the use of faecal microbiota transplantation and emerging therapeutic indications. The Lancet. 2019 Aug 3;394(10196):420-431.

[24] Tang G, Yin W, Liu W. Is frozen fecal microbiota transplantation as effective as fresh fecal microbiota transplantation in patients with recurrent or refractory Clostridium difficile infection: a meta-analysis?. Diagnostic microbiology and infectious disease. 2017 Aug 1;88(4):322-329.

[25] Kao D, Roach B, Silva M, Beck P, Rioux K, Kaplan GG, Chang HJ, Coward S, Goodman KJ, Xu H, Madsen K. Effect of oral capsule–vs colonoscopy-delivered fecal microbiota transplantation on recurrent Clostridium difficile infection: a randomized clinical trial. Jama. 2017 Nov 28;318(20):1985-1993.

[26] Cammarota G, Ianiro G, Tilg H, Rajilić-Stojanović M, Kump P, Satokari R, Sokol H, Arkkila P, Pintus C, Hart A, Segal J. European consensus conference on faecal microbiota transplantation in clinical practice. Gut. 2017 Apr 1;66(4):569-580.

[27] Emanuelsson F, Claesson BE, Ljungström L, Tvede M, Ung KA. Faecal microbiota transplantation and bacteriotherapy for recurrent Clostridium difficile infection: a retrospective evaluation of 31 patients. Scandinavian journal of infectious diseases. 2014 Feb 1;46(2):89-97.

[28] Mattila E, Uusitalo–Seppälä R, Wuorela M, Lehtola L, Nurmi H, Ristikankare M, Moilanen V, Salminen K, Seppälä M, Mattila PS, Anttila VJ. Fecal transplantation,

through colonoscopy, is effective therapy for recurrent Clostridium difficile infection. Gastroenterology. 2012 Mar 1;142(3):490-496.

[29] Rossen NG, MacDonald JK, de Vries EM, D'Haens GR, de Vos WM, Zoetendal EG, Ponsioen CY. Fecal microbiota transplantation as novel therapy in gastroenterology: a systematic review. World journal of gastroenterology: WJG. 2015 May 7;21(17):5359.

[30] Marcella C, Cui B, Kelly CR, Ianiro G, Cammarota G, Zhang F. Systematic review: the global incidence of faecal microbiota transplantation-related adverse events from 2000 to 2020. Alimentary Pharmacology & Therapeutics. 2020 Nov 7.

[31] Kahn SA, Gorawara-Bhat R, Rubin DT. Fecal bacteriotherapy for ulcerative colitis: patients are ready, are we?. Inflammatory bowel diseases. 2012 Apr 1;18(4):676-684.

[32] Bunnik EM, Aarts N, Chen LA. Physicians must discuss potential long-term risks of fecal microbiota transplantation to ensure informed consent. The American Journal of Bioethics. 2017 May 4;17(5):61-63.

[33] Turnbaugh PJ, Ley RE, Mahowald MA, Magrini V, Mardis ER, Gordon JI. An obesity-associated gut microbiome with increased capacity for energy harvest. nature. 2006 Dec;444(7122):1027.

[34] Bercik P, Denou E, Collins J, Jackson W, Lu J, Jury J, Deng Y, Blennerhassett P, Macri J, McCoy KD, Verdu EF. The intestinal microbiota affect central levels of brain-derived neurotropic factor and behavior in mice. Gastroenterology. 2011 Aug 1;141(2):599-609.

[35] Long C, Yu Y, Cui B, et al. A novel quick transendoscopic enteral tubing in mid-gut: technique and training with video. BMC Gastroenterol. 2018;18:37.

[36] Ekekezie C, Perler BK, Wexler A, Duff C, Lillis CJ, Kelly CR. Understanding the scope of do-it-yourself fecal microbiota transplant. Am J Gastroenterol. 2020;115: 603-607.

[37] Cottone M, Pietrosi G, Martorana G, Casa A, Pecoraro G, Oliva L, Orlando A, Rosselli M, Rizzo A, Pagliaro L. Prevalence of cytomegalovirus infection in severe refractory ulcerative and Crohn's colitis. The American journal of gastroenterology. 2001 Mar 1;96(3):773-775.

[38] Bunnik EM, Janssens AC, Schermer MH. A tiered-layered-staged model for informed consent in personal genome testing. European Journal of Human Genetics. 2013 Jun;21(6):596-601.

[39] Schwartz JA. Innovation in pediatric surgery: the surgical innovation continuum and the ETHICAL model. Journal of Pediatric Surgery. 2014 Apr 1;49(4):639-645.

[40] Broekman ML, Carrière ME, Bredenoord AL. Surgical innovation: the ethical agenda: a systematic review. Medicine. 2016 Jun;95(25).

[41] Ye ZN, Xia HH, Zhang R, Li L, Wu LH, Liu XJ, Xie WR, He XX. The Efficacy of Washed Microbiota Transplantation on Helicobacter pylori Eradication: A Pilot Study. Gastroenterology Research and Practice. 2020 Oct 19;2020.

[42] Zhang T, Lu G, Zhao Z, Liu Y, Shen Q, Li P, Chen Y, Yin H, Wang H, Marcella C, Cui B. Washed microbiota transplantation vs. manual fecal microbiota transplantation: clinical findings, animal studies and in vitro screening. Protein & Cell. 2020 Jan 9:1-6.

[43] Fecal Microbiota Transplantation-standardization Study Group. Nanjing consensus on methodology of washed microbiota transplantation. Chinese medical journal. 2020 Oct 5;133(19):2330-2332.

[44] Ianiro G, Mullish BH, Kelly CR, Kassam Z, Kuijper EJ, Ng SC, Iqbal TH, Allegretti JR, Bibbò S, Sokol H, Zhang F. Reorganisation of faecal microbiota transplant services during the COVID-19 pandemic. Gut. 2020 Sep 1;69(9):1555-1563.

[45] https://www.fda.gov/safety/medical-product-safety-information/fecal-microbiota-transplantation-new-safety-information-regarding-additional-protections-screening

[46] Allen J, Sears CL. Impact of the gut microbiome on the genome and epigenome of colon epithelial cells: contributions to colorectal cancer development. Genome medicine. 2019 Dec 1;11(1):11.

[47] Dailey FE, Turse EP, Daglilar E, Tahan V. The dirty aspects of fecal microbiota transplantation: a review of its adverse effects and complications. Current opinion in pharmacology. 2019 Dec 1;49:29-33.

[48] Abu-Sbeih H, Ali FS, Wang Y. Clinical review on the utility of fecal microbiota transplantation in immunocompromised patients. Current gastroenterology reports. 2019 Mar 1;21(3):8.

Chapter 7

Control of Clinical Laboratory Errors by FMEA Model

Hoda Sabati, Amin Mohsenzadeh and Nooshin Khelghati

Abstract

Patient safety is an aim for clinical applications and is a fundamental principle of healthcare and quality management. The main global health organizations have incorporated patient safety in their review of work practices. The data provided by the medical laboratories have a direct impact on patient safety and a fault in any of processes such as strategic, operational and support, could affect it. To provide appreciate and reliable data to the physicians, it is important to emphasize the need to design risk management plan in the laboratory. Failure Mode and Effect Analysis (FMEA) is an efficient technique for error detection and reduction. Technical Committee of the International Organization for Standardization (ISO) licensed a technical specification for medical laboratories suggesting FMEA as a method for prospective risk analysis of high-risk processes. FMEA model helps to identify quality failures, their effects and risks with their reduction/elimination, which depends on severity, probability and detection. Applying FMEA in clinical approaches can lead to a significant reduction of the risk priority number (RPN).

Keywords: Patient Safety, Medical Laboratory, Risks, Failure Modes, Processes

1. Introduction

All medical cares, including clinical laboratories, carries an intrinsic risk of errors that can result in harm, disability, and even death so today their activities have seen a significant increase in monitoring [1]. In the past, laboratory processes performed in clinical laboratories focused only on results, while today, they focus on issues related to reliability, safety and effectiveness. It is very important in health world, being aware of the error rate attributable to health system that has great impact on patients [2]. Currently, some strategies are proposed to analyze and to see how you can decline the rate of preventable errors. In order to guarantee reliable results and improved data consistency, while operating with reduced funding, laboratories need to acquire a new culture of management, more tools and specific training [3]. Research management founded on a quality approach is emerging as an essential tool to ensure valuable, vigorous and dependable consequences, within a framework of the best practice. Risk management has been disseminated in clinical laboratories only for the last years, although it has been applied in healthcare since the 80s. That was partly due to constant inspections during the cycle of laboratory examination, rework, removal of any defects and adjustment after the identification of possible causes of flaws or errors. One of the instruments used in risk management is the analysis of failure modes and effects analysis (FMEA). The FMEA model has been applied in various medical fields, including clinical laboratory activities to improve patient safety before serious harm to their health. By reducing/eliminating errors, the FMEA model helps to prevent and control failures and their risks in clinical approaches [4].

2. Failure mode and effect analysis: background and description

Failure mode and effect analysis (FMEA) which was first developed in the 1940s is a systematic technique for identifying all possible errors in a system or process. Adoption of this analysis by National Aeronautics and Space Administration (NASA) in relation with aerospace missions in mid-1960s made its practical application possible. Since then, this analysis has been widely used in diverse industries such as oil and gas, food and automotive and electronics systems. In recent years FMEA has been also successfully applied in the health system as an effective tool for improving patient safety and performance in hospitals. Today, The FMEA is emerging as a tool for assessing the risk of clinical trial processes and clinical analytical methods. However, there are still too few reports about this last use and even fewer data are available on the application of the methodology in clinical laboratories [5–8]. The risk assessment in this technique involves identification of potential errors, determining the severity (S), occurrence (O) and effects of each error and reviewing the control actions implemented to prevent or detect (D) errors [9] (**Figure 1**). In the traditional FMEA, to measure these criteria, a numeric scale of 1 to 10 is used (**Table 1**). Thus, each failure mode is been ranked by a scale called Risk Priority Number (RPN) characterized by multiplying the numbers of three criteria (S, O, D) together. Therefore, the higher the RPN value, the more important the error is and its correction has more priority. So, RPN is so beneficial to identify high risk failures modes requiring priority functions [10, 11].

Prevention, reducing or excluding of errors and their risk is an essential requirement in clinical analytical tests which is been established by the laboratory according to RPN limit. The laboratory decided the assessing scale of frequency, the severity and errors detection which is being different for each test. There are three main categories of errors [12, 13]:

I. Critical errors – Mainly through request for analysis, if not identified and corrected early, have serious consequences for the patient's health

II. Major errors – resulting from the inappropriate application of the sampling method

III. Minor errors – considered so, because of the low probability of occurrence, the high probability of detection or low/absent severity. These errors are taken into account only with the purpose to review the method and the technical instruction

Classification of potential errors occurred in the clinical laboratory processes which are subjected to the samples shown in **Table 2** (The following items only examples of errors and do and does not include all clinical laboratory failure modes) [14, 15].

In clinical laboratories all errors should be controlled by quality indicators. To monitor and assess periodically laboratories' involvement in patients' care the implementation of quality indicators is necessary. ISO/TS 22367 supports the non-conformities, errors and incidents identifying in the clinical laboratory, with an emphasis on the pre-analytical and post-analytical processes. These processes are

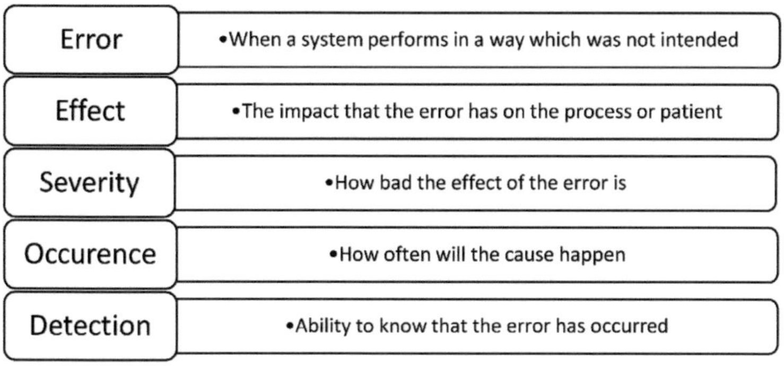

Figure 1.
FMEA elements.

Severity scale (scale 1 [least severe] to 10 [most severe] for each effect)				
Minor (1)	**Low (2,3)**	**Moderate (4-6)**	**High (7,8)**	**Very high (9,10)**
The minor nature of this failure will not have a significant effect on the patient or the choice of treatment	Because of this failure, the patient experiences only a minor injury or a minor discomfort	Failure can lead to patient dissatisfaction, which may include discomfort or failure	Dissatisfaction with the nature of the failure leads to serious disruption and risk to the patient's health	This failure affects safety or increases mortality. This may endanger the patient's life

(I)

Probability scale (scale 1 [least frequent] to 10 [most frequent] for the occurrence)					
Remote (1)	**Very low (2)**	**Low (3,4,5)**	**Moderate (6,7)**	**High (8,9)**	**Very high (10)**
Failure is unlikely; This failure was never observed	Only a few separates failures have ever been observed or reported	Isolated failures have been encountered	Occasional minor failures have been encountered	Failure is often encountered	Failure is almost inevitable

(II)

Detection scale for occurrence (scale 1 [always detected] to 10 [never detected] for each occurrence)					
Very high (1,2)	**High (3,4)**	**Moderate (5,6)**	**Low (7,8)**	**Very low (9)**	**No detection (10)**
It is almost certain to detect the failure mode	There is a good chance of detecting the failure mode	One may detect the existence of the failure mode	There is a poor chance of detecting the existence of the failure mode	One probably will not detect the existence of the failure mode	The existence of the failure mode will not or cannot be detected

(III)

Table 1.
Failure Modes and Effects Analysis Scale for Severity, Probability, and Detection. (I): Severity score (S): 1 to 10 scales from least to most severe (II) Probability score (P): 1 to 10 scales from least to most probable (III) Detectability score (D): 1 to 10 scales from most to least detectable.

Pre-analytical	Analytical	Post-analytical
Incorrect identification of the patient	Procedural non-conformity	Incorrect result
Mislabeling of samples	Errors of equipment or reagents	Result sent to a different patient
Incorrect tube for sampling or incorrect storage	Discrepancies in the results of the internal control	Introducing incorrectly the results in the system
Improper or prolonged transport conditions	Delay in analyzing the samples	Lack of information about the limits concerning the results' interpretation

Table 2.
Potential errors occurred in the clinical laboratory processes.

the most critical and the most difficult ones to control due to involving of various specialists, sections and centers [16]. Clinical laboratory process map is shown in **Figure 2**. The processes map together with the risk map can give us an overview of the failures distribution in each of the processes [3].

Like any analytical method, FMEA should be thoroughly understood prior to being introduced in laboratory practice. There are five stages in its implementation which will be explained in more detail in the methodology [17–19].

FMEA assessment resulted in actions to address the root causes, determining the following situations:

- risk reduction through the development of a preventive action plan to promote process improvement;
- immediate removal of the risk source when the pieces of equipment were increased;
- change in the probability of certain risks when the selection process for new employees was initiated;
- sharing the risk with other staff members when the clinical emergency staff was involved in the potential problem.

FMEA contributed to quality planning, allowing the evaluation of interconnected activities designed to generate products and assisting in the identification of controls.

2.1 FMEA in clinical laboratory activities and patient' safety

Errors in the laboratory activities can lead to consequences in patients' safety. That's why these errors should be identified, controlled and reduced. Effective patient treatment can be improved by prevention and detection of the errors at the time of occurrence which in turn ensures the patient' safety. Currently, the tendency to move from the traditional technical adopted like internal quality control (IQC) and external quality assessment (EQA) to risk management is seen in all quality systems of clinical laboratories. It is conclusive the need for risk management in clinical laboratories and monitoring them within the quality plan, a fact that would lead to an increase on patient safety. Studies have revealed that FMEA is useful for detecting errors and improving patients' safety and it can yield benefits, for failures management and general process improvement, within a laboratory system where

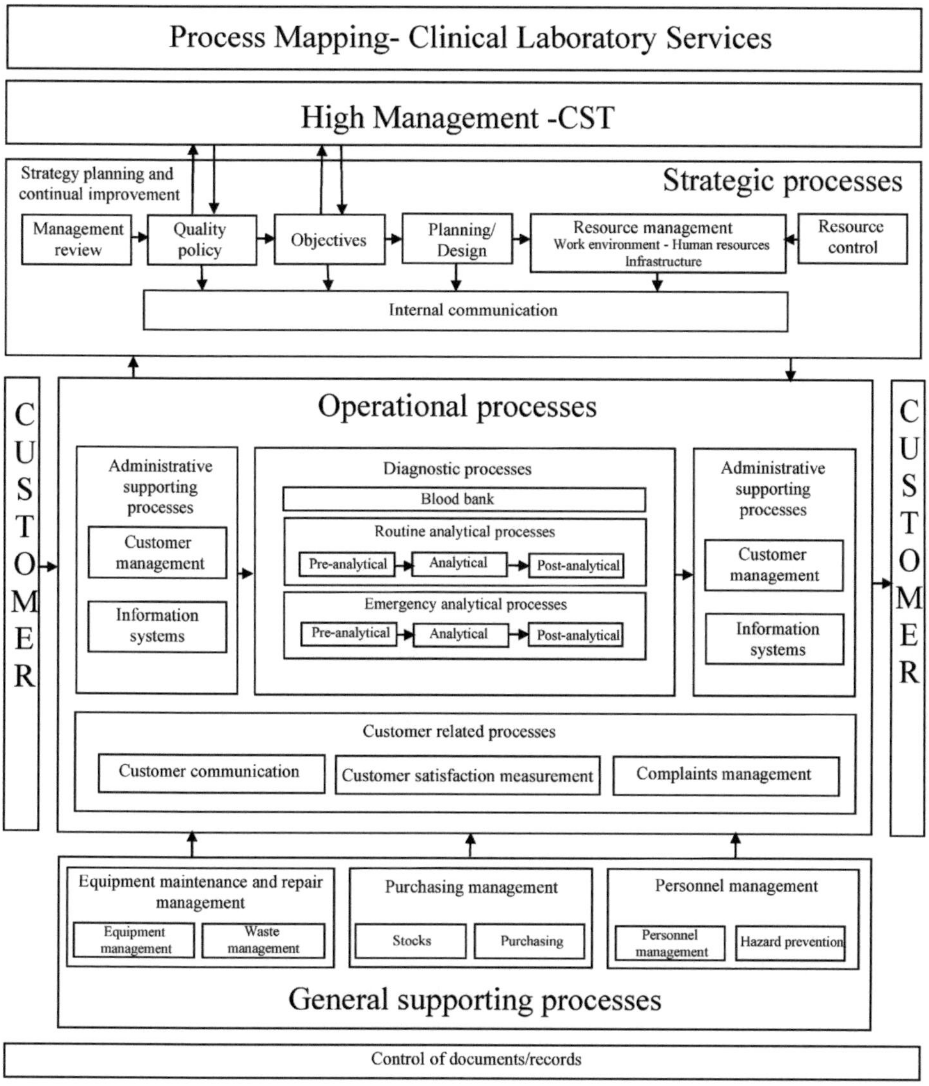

Figure 2.
Processes map of clinical laboratory.

time and team input is limited, and within a process that was considered to have few obstacles [1–4]. Former study showed that FMEA can effectively reduce errors in clinical chemistry laboratories [20].

Woodhouse et al. showed applying FMEA for identified processes in a hemotherapy service, can reduced the possibility of error occurrence and increased the probability of detection [21]. Momenizadeh et al. concluded that implementing FMEA can significantly reduce laboratory errors [22]. Molavi-Taleghani et al. argued that FMEA method is very effective in identifying the possible failure of treatment procedures, determining the cause of each failure mode, and proposing improvement strategies [23]. Applying the FMEA risk assessment tool to laboratory processes can increase effectiveness, efficiency and reproducibility of the results [24]. Risk management in the clinical laboratory by FMEA can decrease the possibility of errors occurrence and ensures the accuracy of results and patient's safety. Risk management guidelines recommended that the clinical laboratories must have a proactive and individualized role in reducing the potential errors by developing an appreciate Quality

Control Plan (QCP). The laboratories must create their own analytic process to identify the weakness of each testing stage. As errors and their risks were identified, the laboratories select the appropriate control processes to detect and to prevent the occurrence of errors. All errors and control processes are mentioned in the QCP [25].

2.2 FMEA benefits and barriers

The Benefits of implementing FMEA approach in clinical laboratories include enhancing patients' safety, improving quality of tests, reducing the chances of repeating the same failure, cost and time and encouragement for teamwork and effective communication between functions – collaboration [26]. In comparison with other quality improvement tools FMEA can be fairly compared, its risk can be assessed, and a score can be assigned.

FMEA also has some barriers such as limits of human error analysis (traditional FMEA uses potential equipment/system failures) and missing interactions between faults and external influences. The reproducibility and generalizability of FMEA in clinical laboratory approaches are factors of concern but since this method is based on hypothetical possibilities uncertainty is still likely to remain [27]. Previous study showed that using FMEA is more time-consuming than other hazard analysis that identifies failure modes but the improvement potentially obtainable by FMEA in a clinical laboratory is high, and this fact should suggest further experiences in this field. Despite the barriers, FMEA represents an appreciate, comprehensive, and organized approach to known potential patient safety failure modes in clinical laboratory [28–30]. processes. According to the *risk-based thinking* introduced by new ISO 9001:2015 standard, FMEA is an appropriate approach errors analysis of operational processes under an ISO-certified Quality Management System [31].

3. Methodology

Analytical methodology of FMEA is very effective in maintaining patient safety. Laboratory staffs trained in FMEA methodology can greatly reduce time requirements and guarantee that all activities involved are coordinated increasing the accuracy of laboratory results [17–19].

The FMEA process including 5 steps as follow:

1. Selecting a process for study;
2. Assembling a multidisciplinary team;
3. Collecting and organizing data about the selected process;
4. Analysis of hazards;
5. Developing and implementing appropriate actions and measuring the outcomes;

3.1 Selecting a process for study

The intricacy of laboratory processes increases the probability of undesirable errors. The more steps in the process and the greater their dependency, the greater the chance of error. In this step the laboratory identifies the critical processes based on the severity of possible harmful errors and the potentially dangerous impact on patient safety [17–19].

3.2 Assembling a multidisciplinary team

Gathering specialists with different levels and types of training, with specific knowledge and experience of the selected process. A team head can lead team members through the process, and can help ensure that team members complete each step and record the results of FMEA [17–19].

3.3 Collecting and organizing data about the selected process

In this step the assembled team creates an accurate diagram of potential failure modes of each listed activity using focus laboratory staff activities and reaching a common conclusion and recording it on FMEA form (**Table 3**) [17–19].

3.4 Analysis of hazards

This step including identifying failure modes in each step, determining the potential effect of each failure mode, ranking the severity of failure mode effects, ranking the probability and detectability of each failure mode and identifying the critical failure modes [17–19].

3.5 Developing and implementing appropriate actions and measuring the outcomes

Identifying the root causes of critical failures is an important step in developing an appropriate action plan. Traditional root cause analysis methods are used to

Project: **Product:** **System:**					**Date:** **Prepared by:**					**FMEA number:** **Reference documents:**	
System Component Function	Potential failure mode	Potential consequences/effects of failure	Severity	Critical	Potential causes of failure	Probability	Current design controls	Detection	RPN	Recommended actions	Responsibility And completion date

Table 3.
FMEA form.

determine the underlying cause of each critical failure so that appropriate actions can be taken. Once the root causes of critical failures have been identified, the team's aim is to eliminate the risk of failures, reduce the likelihood of failure or mitigate the effects of failure should it affect the patient [17–19].

4. Discussion

Clinical laboratories processes tend to errors due to human interactions and instrumental mistakes. Therefore, it is essential to design plans to make errors preventable. In the clinical laboratory, most errors are in the pre-analytical phase. The criteria for risk assessment designing plans for preventive errors were defined in the laboratory. There is no standard for developing and implementing of these plans in the laboratory, impediment the comparison between pairs and application of best practices. Some of the staff laboratory features, namely the ability to think analytical and simultaneously to establish standard policies and strict adherence to protocols, helped in the prevention of the potential errors. These plans for risk assessment can help reduce the occurrence of adverse errors. FMEA may become the common standard for measurement and comparison, particularly in clinical laboratories. In fact, the total testing process is intricate, consisting of numerous steps that are not always taken under the control of laboratory experts. Current evidence on the stratification of errors in clinical laboratory strongly supports the introduction of FMEA for further reducing error rates, particularly in the extra-analytical steps. While the first aim of FMEA is to promote an approach to ensuring the safety of laboratory processes, total cost reduction should be simultaneously achieved when considering the entire process of patient safety [13–16].

Mascia et al. shows that the FMEA risk management approach as applied to a scientific processes is in line with the current needs of management models to raise effectiveness and efficiency, to enhance reproducibility, and to facilitate a rapid industrialization of obtained results [24]. In order to achieve reliable results in long run of clinical laboratory approaches Momenizadeh et al. suggested that the managers of the laboratories of Markazi province (Iran) should focus on the implementation of the FMEA [22]. Sudhakar et al. reported that FMEA is a beneficial technique to decrease quality failures in clinical biochemistry laboratories. As compared to other prospective risk analysis approaches, FMEA prevent and solve high risk failure modes in clinical laboratories [32]. Previous study stated the efficiency of FMEA risk assessment to detect and to adjust the quality control procedures in order to improve the analytical performance of clinical chemistry laboratories [33].

In all clinical laboratories a risk assessment approach is required according to ISO 17025:2017 standard dedicated to laboratories measurement, in order to improve uncertainty and thus the reliability and reproducibility of results. Performing FMEA to processes in the laboratory facilitates evaluation high-risk processes tend to failure before an error happen. By assuming and compensating for less-than-perfect human performance, FMEA promotes error prevention through identification of valuable and consensually accepted quality indicators in all steps of the testing process [34].

5. Conclusion

Clinical laboratories are inseparable part of health care system as they help in appropriate diagnosis of patient's health. Their working process is a complex procedure which may associate with certain errors. Improvement of the patients' safety by reducing the errors and their risks in clinical laboratories is a great challenge. High-quality clinical laboratories ensure that they perform standard tasks, monitor, and improve their performance, creating a culture of transparency, defining responsibilities, and optimizing patients' safety. FMEA is very effective and successful technique in preventing errors, improving quality and safety of tests, identifying potential errors, and prioritizing clinical laboratory improvement strategies. FMEA had a multidisciplinary approach and its complex configuration processes involvement facilitated the management of errors. As compared to other prospective risk analysis methods, FMEA analysis provides a good solution for high risk failure modes in clinical laboratories. Therefore, FMEA is a suitable and efficient tool to identify most clinical laboratory errors to improving the quality of laboratory processes and ensuring the accuracy of obtained results and maintaining patient health and safety. The overall purpose of this paper is to encourage clinical laboratories to assess and monitor their own. In addition, it should be possible to identify and monitor error rates to improve upon the process on the basis of objective and desirable quality specifications.

Conflict of interests

The authors declare that they have no conflicts of interest.

Author contributions

All authors contributed equally to this manuscript, and approved the final version of manuscripts.

Ethical declarations

Not applicable.

Financial support

None to be declared.

Author details

Hoda Sabati[1*], Amin Mohsenzadeh[2] and Nooshin Khelghati[3]

1 Faculty of Science, Biotechnology and Biological Science Research Center, Shahid Chamran University of Ahvaz, Ahvaz, Iran

2 Faculty of Science, Department of Microbiology, Ardabil Branch, Islamic Azad University, Ardabil, Iran

3 Faculty of Science, Department of Chemistry, Shahid Chamran University of Ahvaz, Ahvaz, Iran

*Address all correspondence to: h.sabati@yahoo.com

References

[1] Kalra, J. (2011). *Medical errors and patient safety: strategies to reduce and disclose medical errors and improve patient safety* (Vol. 1). Walter de Gruyter.

[2] Plebani, M. (2010). The detection and prevention of errors in laboratory medicine. *Annals of clinical biochemistry*, *47*(2), 101-110.

[3] Lao, E. G., García, Á. S., Figuerola, M. B., Moreno, E., & Paraire, A. H. (2017). Errors of clinical laboratory and its impact on patient safety. *Open Journal of Social Sciences*, *5*(3), 243-253.

[4] Mascia, A., Cirafici, A. M., Bongiovanni, A., Colotti, G., Lacerra, G., Di Carlo, M., ... & Kisslinger, A. (2020). A failure mode and effect analysis (FMEA)-based approach for risk assessment of scientific processes in non-regulated research laboratories. *Accreditation and Quality Assurance*, *25*(5), 311-321.

[5] Sharma, K. D., & Srivastava, S. (2018). Failure mode and effect analysis (FMEA) implementation: a literature review. *J Adv Res Aeronaut Space Sci*, *5*, 2454-8669.

[6] Banduka, N., Veža, I., & Bilić, B. (2016). An integrated lean approach to Process Failure Mode and Effect Analysis (PFMEA): A case study from automotive industry. *Advances in Production Engineering & Management*, *11*(4).

[7] Yusof, M. B., & Abdullah, N. H. B. (2016). Failure mode and effect analysis (FMEA) of butterfly valve in oil and gas industry. *J. Eng. Sci. Technol.*, *11*, 9-19.

[8] Goel, A., & Graves, R. J. (2007, May). Using failure mode effect analysis to increase electronic systems reliability. In *2007 30th International Spring Seminar on Electronics Technology (ISSE)* (pp. 128-133). IEEE.

[9] Chiozza, M. L., & Ponzetti, C. (2009). FMEA: a model for reducing medical errors. *Clinica chimica acta*, *404*(1), 75-78.

[10] Rezaei, F., Yarmohammadian, M. H., Haghshenas, A., Fallah, A., & Ferdosi, M. (2018). Revised risk priority number in failure mode and effects analysis model from the perspective of healthcare system. *International journal of preventive medicine*, *9*.

[11] Liu, H. C. (2019). *Improved FMEA methods for proactive healthcare risk analysis*. Singapore: Springer.

[12] Mendes, M. E., Ebner, P. D. A. R., Romano, P., Pacheco Neto, M., Sant'anna, A., & Sumita, N. M. (2013). Practical aspects of the use of FMEA tool in clinical laboratory risk management. *Jornal Brasileiro de Patologia e Medicina Laboratorial*, *49*(3), 174-181.

[13] Marin, A. G., Rivas-Ruiz, F., del Mar Pérez-Hidalgo, M., & Molina-Mendoza, P. (2014). Pre-analytical errors management in the clinical laboratory: a five-year study. *Biochemia medica*, *24*(2), 248-257.

[14] Plebani, M. (2006). Errors in clinical laboratories or errors in laboratory medicine. *Clinical Chemistry and Laboratory Medicine (CCLM)*, *44*(6), 750-759.

[15] International Organization for Standardization/Technical Specification. (2008). Medical Laboratories-Reduction of Error Through Risk Management and Continual Improvement. ISO/TS 22367: 2008.

[16] International Organization for Standardization. (2012). *Medical laboratories: requirements for quality and competence*. ISO.

[17] Schmittner, C., Gruber, T., Puschner, P., & Schoitsch, E. (2014, September). Security application of failure mode and effect analysis (FMEA). In *International Conference on Computer Safety, Reliability, and Security* (pp. 310-325). Springer, Cham.

[18] Moradi, L., Emami Sigaroudi, A., Pourshaikhian, M., & Heidari, M. (2020). Risk Assessment of Clinical Care in Emergency Departments by Health Failure Modes and Effects Analysis. *Journal of Holistic Nursing and Midwifery*, *30*(1), 35-44.

[19] Thornton, E., Brook, O. R., Mendiratta-Lala, M., Hallett, D. T., & Kruskal, J. B. (2011). Application of failure mode and effect analysis in a radiology department. *Radiographics*, *31*(1), 281-293.

[20] Jiang, Y., Jiang, H., Ding, S., & Liu, Q. (2015). Application of failure mode and effects analysis in a clinical chemistry laboratory. *Clinica Chimica Acta*, *448*, 80-85.

[21] Woodhouse, S., Burney, B., & Coste, K. (2004). To err is human: improving patient safety through failure mode and effect analysis. *Clinical leadership & management review: the journal of CLMA*, *18*(1), 32-36.

[22] Momenizadeh, E., Riahi, L., & Nazarimanesh, L. (2019). The effect of controlling clinical laboratory errors on patients' safety in Markazi province laboratories. *Razi Journal of Medical Sciences*, *26*(9), 102-111.

[23] Molavi-Taleghani, Y., Ebrahimpour, H., & Sheikhbardsiri, H. (2020). A Proactive Risk Assessment Through Healthcare Failure Mode and Effect Analysis in Pediatric Surgery Department. *Journal of Comprehensive Pediatrics*, *11*(3).

[24] Mascia, A., Cirafici, A. M., Bongiovanni, A., Colotti, G., Lacerra, G., Di Carlo, M., ... & Kisslinger, A. (2020). A failure mode and effect analysis (FMEA)-based approach for risk assessment of scientific processes in non-regulated research laboratories. *Accreditation and Quality Assurance*, *25*(5), 311-321.

[25] Eliza, D. R., & Minodora, D. (2015). Risk Management in Clinical Laboratory: from Theory to Practice. *Acta Medica Marisiensis*, *61*(4), 372-377.

[26] Tosheska-Trajkovska, K., Bosilkova, G., Kostovska, I., Labudovikj, D., Brezovska Kavrakova, J., Cekovska, S., ... & Marija, K. (2019). Risk management in the clinical laboratories-use of the Failure Modes and Effects Analysis (FMEA). *Journal of Morphological Sciences*.

[27] Stravitz, P. E., Cibas, E. S., & Heher, Y. K. (2019). Targeting specimen misprocessing safety events with failure modes and effects analysis. *Cancer cytopathology*, *127*(4), 213-217.

[28] Mendes, M. E., Ebner, P. D. A. R., Romano, P., Pacheco Neto, M., Sant'anna, A., & Sumita, N. M. (2013). Practical aspects of the use of FMEA tool in clinical laboratory risk management. *Jornal Brasileiro de Patologia e Medicina Laboratorial*, *49*(3), 174-181.

[29] David, R. E., & Dobreanu, M. I. N. O. D. O. R. A. (2015). Failure modes and effects analysis (FMEA)-An assessment tool for risk management in clinical laboratories. *Acta Medica Transilvanica*, *20*(4), 130-34.

[30] Potts, H. W., Anderson, J. E., Colligan, L., Leach, P., Davis, S., & Berman, J. (2014). Assessing the validity of prospective hazard analysis methods: a comparison of two techniques. *BMC health services research*, *14*(1), 1-10.

[31] Corpuz, R. S. A. (2020). ISO 9001: 2015 Risk-based Thinking: A Framework

using Fuzzy-Support Vector Machine. *Makara Journal of Technology*, *24*(3), 149-159.

[32] Sudhakar, B., & Sadariya, B. R. (2020). Application of failure mode and effects analysis to minimize quality failures in clinical biochemistry laboratory. *International Journal of Clinical Biochemistry and Research*, *5*(4), 613-616.

[33] Xia, Y., Xue, H., Yan, C., Li, B., Zhang, S., Li, M., & Ji, L. (2018). Risk analysis and assessment based on Sigma metrics and intended use. *Biochemia medica*, *28*(2), 195-203.

[34] Vasilnakova, A. (2018). RISK MANAGEMENT IN ACCREDITED TESTING LABORATORIES. Annals of DAAAM & Proceedings, 29.

Chapter 8

Specialized Training for Nursing in the Surgical Area, a Question of Quality

María Desamparados Bernat Adell, María Sánchez Galán, Ana Folch Ayora, Pablo Salas Molina and Eladio Joaquín Collado Boira

Abstract

This is an observational, descriptive and cross-sectional study that looks into nursing competencies within the surgical area and analyzes the influence of the variables age, years worked and employment relationship on the dependent variable nursing competencies. The Perceived Perioperative Competence Scale-Revised (PPCS-R) questionnaire was applied to nurses in the surgical area of the General University Hospital of Castellón. The variables were processed using ANOVA tests and Pearson's correlations. A sample of 50 female nurses with a mean age of 41 ± 7.931 years was evaluated. Age and number of years worked were positively related to 11 items of the questionnaire. Regarding the employment relationship, significant differences were found, with the "permanent" employment relationship obtaining the highest mean score [1.040 ($p = .018$)]. Education and clinical experience were found to contribute to the development of practice. Patient safety was an essential aspect in managing the associated risk in the operating room (OR).

Keywords: competence, clinical experience, specialized competence, specialized education, surgical area

1. Introduction

The nursing discipline has undergone constant development, both at a conceptual and at a theoretical and practical level. The minimum academic level to obtain the basic competencies is the University Degree in Nursing, which is based on the regulations of the European Higher Education Area (EHEA), which, in turn, provide a solid base in the sciences of behavior, life and care and open the possibility of creating ascending levels of academic recognition within the same discipline: degree, masters and doctorate [1].

Academic nursing degree programs certify the possession of foundational competencies. In some areas of nursing knowledge, there is the possibility of focusing training after obtaining the degree towards a more specialized field that allows the professional to perform better in situations of greater complexity [2].

In Spain, this specialized training has undergone a development parallel to that of the nursing discipline. The Law 44/2003, of the 21st of November, on the organization of the health professions included, for the first time, the specific definition and catalog of nursing specialties [3]. The aforementioned catalog was modified by the Royal Decree 450/2005, finally leaving seven specialties: Obstetric-Gynecological Nursing, Mental Health Nursing, Geriatric Nursing, Occupational Health Nursing, Family and Community Nursing, Pediatric Nursing and Medical-Surgical Care Nursing [4]. All the specialties have their own legally supported training program regulated by a residency system (Resident Nursing Intern, Enfermero Interno Residente-EIR in Spanish), except for the Medical-Surgical Care specialty, which is paralyzed due to unknown reasons [5].

Postgraduate training implies the acquisition of competencies inherent to a specific context and nursing specialties guide the professional towards clinically relevant competencies [6, 7]. Consequently, they become a challenge for the profession, which involves combining patient care with highly technical aspects without affecting patient safety [8, 9].

The perioperative setting is dynamic in nature and depends on both knowledge, and clinical judgment and reasoning skills. Therefore, it is an environment that requires specific training, and this becomes a way to provide the highest quality of care, as well as being an essential element in the identification and prevention of errors [10]. Specialized training in surgical areas ensures patient safety and is the cornerstone of clinical practice [11]. A clear description and identification of nursing competencies in the surgical field would make it easier for nurses working in these areas to be specialists with a formally acquired education [6].

It is difficult to completely eliminate the risk associated with healthcare assistance, but awareness should be raised about the professionals' need to acquire specific skills for the prevention of errors and avoidable adverse events, in order to guarantee the safety of the patient and respect their rights. Regulated training, experience and professionalism are considered essential elements for risk management in surgical care [6, 8, 12].

The general objective of the present study is to observe the necessary nursing competencies within the surgical area. It is also intended to observe whether these competencies are modified according to age and sex, the number of years worked and the contractual relationship of the nurses.

2. Methods

This is an observational, descriptive and cross-sectional study, carried out in the Surgical Area of the General University Hospital of Castellón (HGUCS). The target population consisted of all the nurses working in the HGUCS surgical area. At the time of study, there were 87 nurses and 2 supervisors (N = 89). From this population, the study's sample was calculated, taking into account a confidence level of 95% and a margin of error of 3%, accepting a value of statistical significance $p \leq .05$. The studied sample consisted of 62 nurses. Only 50 nurses were interviewed because of the safety measures adopted to prevent the intra-hospital transmission of SARS-CoV-2.

The inclusion criteria were working in the surgical area and being in active service at the time of the study. The only exclusion criterion was the fact that the professional did not wish to participate in the study.

The dependent variables were those provided by the Perceived Perioperative Competence Scale-Revised (PPCS-R) questionnaire applied to assess nursing competencies.

The following were included as independent variables: sociodemographic variables (age and sex) and variables related to work (employment relationship, defined as: permanent contract, indefinite contract and/or temporary contract) and years worked in a surgical area (less than one year, between 1 and 5 years, between 6 and 10 years, and more than 10 years).

The Perceived Perioperative Competence Scale-Revised (PPCS-R) was used, which quantifies both domains of general competence and domains of specific competence. It is a specific self-assessment tool, used to reflect on areas of strengths and limitations within the surgical context [2]. This questionnaire is based on a self-assessment applied through a Likert scale, ranging between 1 and 5, (1 never, 2 sometimes, 3 often, 4 very often, 5 always) with 40 closed-choice questions that address six domains. These domains are foundational knowledge and skills, leadership, collaboration, proficiency, empathy, and professional development. The calculated response time was 20 minutes. The data were collected between the 24th of February and the 13th of March 2020.

2.1 Statistical analyses

The data were processed using the Statistical Package for the Social Sciences (SPSS) v.23.0 statistical program, accepting a level of statistical significance of $p \leq 0.05$.

Regarding the analyses techniques, the description of the characteristics of the sample was carried out by calculating the mean and the standard deviation for the quantitative variables; qualitative variables were expressed in percentages and frequencies. To respond to the specific objectives, the Pearson correlation and the ANOVA test were applied, together with the Scheffé test.

2.2 Ethical considerations

The project was approved as of March 10, 2020 by the HGUCS Clinical Research Committee and the Nursing Directorate.

The participation of the nurses in the study was voluntary. The necessary measures were taken to preserve the confidentiality of personal data in compliance with the Organic Law 3/2018, of the 5th December, on the Protection of Personal Data and Guarantee of digital rights [13] and the declaration of Helsinki [14]. The participants were aware of their right to abandon said study at any given time.

Any personal data that could identify the professional was not used; hence the data collection notebooks were assigned a random number. The paper records were destroyed after being computerized. The study did not receive any public or private funding and the authors declare that they have no conflict of interest.

3. Results

A total of 50 questionnaires were collected ($n = 50$). The mean age of the participants was 41 ± 7.931 years, ranging between 27 and 59 years. The entire sample was composed of women.

Regarding the employment relationship, 22% (11) had a permanent contract, 56% (28) had indefinite contracts, and the remaining 22% (11) had temporary contracts. Regarding the number of years worked, 62% (31) had more than 10 years worked in the surgical area, 12% (6) had between 6 and 10 years, 20% (10) had between 1 and 5 years and 6% (3) had less than 1 year worked in the surgical area.

The descriptive results of the "Perceived Perioperative Competence Scale-Revised" (PPCS-R) questionnaire are presented structured in the six dimensions of the scale. These dimensions are divided into technical and non-technical competencies. Technical competencies include the knowledge and skills dimension, as well as the proficiency dimension. In turn, non-technical competencies are composed of the remaining four dimensions: leadership, collaboration, empathy, and professional development.

Table 1 shows the results of both the "Foundational knowledge and skills" dimension and the "Proficiency" dimension. Regarding the "Foundational knowledge and skills" dimension, it should be noted that the lowest score was obtained by Item number 1 (3.21 ± 1.148), which referred to the variability of surgical instrumentation. Regarding the "Proficiency" dimension, the worst evaluated item was number 29 (3.58 ± 0.835), which dealt with the ability to anticipate the needs that may arise in an intervention. See **Table 1**.

Foundational knowledge and skills		**Proficiency**	
Items	**Mean (SD)**	**Items**	**Mean (SD)**
1. I am familiar with most of the instrumentation in different specialties	3.21 (1.148)	10. I have mastered the terminology and vocabulary of OR nursing	3.90 (.853)
2. I know where to find equipment and supplies in the OR	3.88 (.940)	11. I troubleshoot and take appropriate action in the event of machine/equipment failures	3.82 (.941)
3. My local knowledge of this department assists me to perform my OR role	4.02 (1.078)		
4. I understand and anticipate the surgical procedure	3.58 (.906)	12. Based on experience, I am able to identify actual or potential emergency situations and respond appropriately	4.12 (.799)
5. I am familiar with the technological equipment used in the OR	3.88 (.961)		
6. When I am allocated to an area of the OR that is unfamiliar, I draw on my skills and experience.	3.82 (1.014)	13. I apply specialist knowledge in providing care for OR patients	4.00 (.904)
7. I plan and coordinate the needs in the theater I am allocated	4.02 (.934)	14. I have the right amount of knowledge to practice in this specialty	3.61 (.975)
8. I know instinctively when surgery is not going well and am able to respond appropriately	3.76 (.969)		
9. Knowing the location of equipment in the OR assists me to perform my OR role	4.39 (.812)	15. I am able to anticipate the needs of the situation	3.58 (.835)

Mean: Value of the arithmetic mean. Standard deviation (SD).

Table 1.
Dimensions: Foundational knowledge and skills and proficiency.

In relation to the non-technical competencies, it should be noted that the items in the "Leadership" dimension, in general, have been those that have obtained the lowest ratings; highlighting the mean value (2.64 ± .987) of the item that deals with the ability of a nurse to handle conflict situations among the staff of an operating room. However, nurses have shown interest in cooperating to train novel nurses.

Regarding the "Collaboration" dimension, it is observed that, in general, all the items have higher mean values with a trend approaching 5 as the highest score. In addition, Item 21 shows the respect that nurses have towards more experienced colleagues (4.64 ± .563, see **Table 2**).

Table 3 shows the results of the non-technical competencies "Empathy" and "Professional Development". All the items that are part of the "Empathy" dimension have obtained values close to 5. Perhaps the item that deals with the relationship with patients to make it easier for them to express feelings and concerns, scoring a (4.02 ± .750), points out where training would be required. Regarding the "Professional development" dimension, it is worth highlighting that the lowest valued item (2.90 ± 1.026) is the one that deals with updating knowledge by reading articles, see **Table 3**.

To observe the correlation between age and perioperative competencies, 3 age ranges were established (25 to 40 years, 41 to 50 years and more than 50 years of age). The results of the Pearson correlation indicate the presence of a positive statistically significant correlation for 11 items of the questionnaire; these items were better evaluated with increasing age. See **Table 4**.

All participants were women; therefore, the sex variable was not processed as it was a constant. **Table 5** presents the results of the correlation between "Years

Leadership		**Collaboration**	
Items	**Mean (SD)**	**Items**	**Mean (SD)**
1. I take a leadership role to ensure the smooth running of the theater	2.90 (.984)	9. I use appropriate methods of communication according to the needs of the situation	3.78 (.815)
2. I make difficult decisions when necessary	3.13 (1.104)	10. I feel comfortable in seeking assistance from my colleagues when I am unsure	4.39 (.731)
3. I take an active role in preceptoring or mentoring lesser experienced nurses	3.47 (1.157)		
4. I manage clinical situations when there is conflict between staff	2.64 (.987)	11. I tailor my communication based on the mix of personalities in the team	3.86 (.783)
5. I provide clinical guidance to other staff members	2.90 (1.046)	12. I respect the level of expertise of other members of the team	4.64 (.563)
6. I encourage team members to use innovative solutions to solve traditional problems	2.90 (1.065)	13. I treat members as individuals who have different needs, abilities and aspirations	4.32 (.794)
7. I delegate aspects of care according to role, functions, capabilities and learning needs of other team members	3.06 (1.008)	14. When communicating with other team members, I use language that is appropriate to the situation	4.28 (.607)
8. I encourage active involvement in clinical decision-making processes	2.96 (0,978)		

Mean: Value of the arithmetic mean. Standard deviation (SD).

Table 2.
Dimensions: Leadership and collaboration.

Empathy		Professional development	
Items	**Mean (SD)**	**Items**	**Mean (SD)**
1. I provide reassurance for patients using verbal and non-verbal strategies	4.14 (.791)	35. I maintain current knowledge of, and incorporate relevant organizational policies into practice	3.57 (.866)
2. I use strategies to make the patient feel more comfortable	4.31 (.769)	36. I have detailed knowledge of anatomy and physiology	3.41 (.705)
3. I provide appropriate reassurance and explanation for OR patients	4.16 (.825)	37. I maintain knowledge of, and incorporate relevant standards into my practice	3.45 (.914)
4. I actively listen to the patient and significant others to obtain necessary information	4.35 (.597)	38. I read current journals and literature that relate to clinical practice	2.90 (1.026)
5. I establish rapport with patients that enhances their ability to express feelings and concerns	4.02 (.750)	39. I keep up with the technical changes in procedures and equipment	3.51 (.960)
		40. I use available resources to maintain current OR practice	4.00 (.935)

Mean: Value of the arithmetic mean. Standard deviation (SD).

Table 3.
Dimensions: Empathy and professional development.

Items	Pearson (r)	P-Value
1. I am familiar with most of the instrumentation in different specialties	.385	.012*
2. I know where to find equipment and supplies in the OR	.488	.001***
3. My local knowledge of this department assists me to perform my OR role	.455	.002**
4. I understand and anticipate the surgical procedure	.432	.003**
5. I am familiar with the technological equipment used in the OR	.317	.036*
8. I know instinctively when surgery is not going well and am able to respond appropriately	.322	.035*
9. Knowing the location of equipment in the OR assists me to perform my OR role	.374	.014*
10. I take a leadership role to ensure the smooth running of the theater	.366	.016*
24. I have mastered the terminology and vocabulary of OR nursing	.404	.006**
27. I apply specialist knowledge in providing care for OR patients	.370	.013*
36. I have detailed knowledge of anatomy and physiology	.464	.002**

r: Pearson's correlation coefficient. P-value: $p < .05^{*}$, $p < .01^{**}$, $p < .001^{***}$.

Table 4.
Relationship between the age of the participants and the score of the PPCS-R scale.

worked" and the scores of the (PPCS-R) scale. The "Years worked" were distributed into four groups (less than 1 year worked in the surgical area, between 1 and 5 years, between 6 and 10 years, and more than 10 years). The correlations were positive, indicating that the greater the number of years worked, the better the results obtained, see **Table 5**.

Items	Pearson (r)	P-value
1. I am familiar with most of the instrumentation in different specialties	.409	.005**
2. I know where to find equipment and supplies in the OR	.504	.001***
3. My local knowledge of this department assists me to perform my OR role	.464	.001***
4. I understand and anticipate the surgical procedure	.540	.001***
5. I am familiar with the technological equipment used in the OR	.336	.021*
7. I plan and coordinate the needs in the theater I am allocated	.367	.013*
8. I know instinctively when surgery is not going well and am able to respond appropriately	.440	.002**
9. Knowing the location of equipment in the OR assists me to perform my OR role	.376	.010**
11. I make difficult decisions when necessary	.352	.018*
12. I take an active role in preceptoring or mentoring lesser experienced nurses	.528	.001***
13. I manage clinical situations when there is conflict between staff	.567	.001***
14. I provide clinical guidance to other staff members	.428	.003**
15. I encourage team members to use innovative solutions to solve traditional problems	.470	.001***
16. I delegate aspects of care according to role, functions, capabilities and learning needs of other team members	.388	.008**
17. I encourage active involvement in clinical decision-making processes	.472	.001***
20. I tailor my communication based on the mix of personalities in the team	.330	.023*
24. I have mastered the terminology and vocabulary of OR nursing	.553	.001***
25. I troubleshoot and take appropriate action in the event of machine/equipment failures	.471	.001***
27. I apply specialist knowledge in providing care for OR patients	.599	.001***
28. I have the right amount of knowledge to practice in this specialty	.553	.001***
29. I am able to anticipate the needs of the situation	.513	.001***
32. I provide appropriate reassurance and explanation for OR patients	.298	.045*
34. I establish rapport with patients that enhances their ability to express feelings and concerns	.219	.049*
36. I have detailed knowledge of anatomy and physiology	.540	.001***
39. I keep up with the technical changes in procedures and equipment	.435	.002**
40. I use available resources to maintain current OR practice	.540	.001***

r: Pearson's correlation coefficient. P-value: $p < .05^*$, $p < .01^{**}$, $p < .001^{***}$.

Table 5.
Relationship between the years worked and the results in the PPCS-R scale.

The significant results of the ANOVA test that observe whether the means of the scores obtained in the PPCS-R scale presented differences depending on the employment relationship are presented in **Table 6**. See **Table 6**.

Scheffé's test was applied to observe which employment relationship was the one that presented the differences found in the ANOVA test. As a more noteworthy general results, professionals with a permanent employment relationship presented higher mean values and better evaluations on the scale (PPCS-R). See **Table 7**.

Items	F-Value	p-value
2. I know where to find equipment and supplies in the OR	4.231	.021*
3. My local knowledge of this department assists me to perform my OR role	7.608	.001***
4. I understand and anticipate the surgical procedure	6.102	.005**
5. I am familiar with the technological equipment used in the OR	4.315	.020*
6. When I am allocated to an area of the OR that is unfamiliar, I draw on my skills and experience.	4.594	.016*
8. I know instinctively when surgery is not going well and am able to respond appropriately	4.138	.023*
9. Knowing the location of equipment in the OR assists me to perform my OR role	3.996	.026*
24. I have mastered the terminology and vocabulary of OR nursing	7.736	.001***
25. I troubleshoot and take appropriate action in the event of machine/ equipment failures	4.753	.014*
26. Based on experience, I am able to identify actual or potential emergency situations and respond appropriately	6.220	.004**
27. I apply specialist knowledge in providing care for OR patients	6.141	.005**
28. I have the right amount of knowledge to practice in this specialty	6.029	.005**
29. I am able to anticipate the needs of the situation	7.822	.001***
38. I read current journals and literature that relate to clinical practice	4.529	.017*

*F: Coefficient of the ANOVA test. p-value: $p < .05$ *, $p < .01$ **, $p < .001$ ***.*

Table 6.
Differences between employment relationship and the results in the PPCS-R scale.

Items	Employment relationship (I)	Employment relationship (J)	Mean difference (I-J)	p-value
2. I know where to find equipment and supplies in the OR	Permanent	Temporary contract	1.100	.023*
3. My local knowledge of this department assists me to perform my OR role	Permanent	Temporary contract	1.600	.002**
	Indefinite contract	Temporary contract	1.015	.021*
4. I understand and anticipate the surgical procedure	Permanent	Temporary contract	1.200	.005**
5. I am familiar with the technological equipment used in the OR	Permanent	Temporary contract	1.100	.006**
6. When I am allocated to an area of the OR that is unfamiliar, I draw on my skills and experience.	Permanent	Temporary contract	1.200	.025*
	Indefinite contract	Temporary contract	.923	.044*
8. I know instinctively when surgery is not going well and am able to respond appropriately	Indefinite contract	Temporary contract	1.000	.025*
9. Knowing the location of equipment in the OR assists me to perform my OR role	Permanent	Temporary contract	.911	.027*
24. I have mastered the terminology and vocabulary of OR nursing	Permanent	Temporary contract	1.300	.001***

Items	Employment relationship (I)	Employment relationship (J)	Mean difference (I-J)	p-value
25. I troubleshoot and take appropriate action in the event of machine/ equipment failures	Permanent	Temporary contract	1.200	.014*
26. Based on experience, I am able to identify actual or potential emergency situations and respond appropriately	Permanent	Temporary contract	1.000	.008**
	Indefinite contract	Temporary contract	.769	.016*
27. I apply specialist knowledge in providing care for OR patients	Permanent	Temporary contract	1.200	.006**
	Indefinite contract	Temporary contract	.777	.038*
28. I have the right amount of knowledge to practice in this specialty	Permanent	Temporary contract	1.411	.005**
29. I am able to anticipate the needs of the situation	Permanent	Indefinite contract	.700	.031*
	Permanent	Temporary contract	1.200	.001***
38. I read current journals and literature that relate to clinical practice	Permanent	Indefinite contract	1.040	.018*

The differences are presented with a positive sign. (I-J): Scheffé post hoc test. p-value: $p < .05^*$, $p < .01^{**}$, $p < .001^{***}$.

Table 7.
Group differences between employment relationship and results in the PPCS-R scale.

4. Discussion

Stobinski argued in 2008 that which determines what a professional is capable of doing can be expressed in measurable actions, so that assessment in a precise way becomes an essential practice implied in care [15]. We agree that, in a highly specialized clinical context, such as in surgical areas, identifying the nurses' competencies and measuring which variables modify them is necessary.

In our case and using the "Perceived Perioperative Competence Scale-Revised" (PPCS-R) questionnaire, perioperative competencies were evaluated across a total of 50 nurses from the surgical area of the HGUCS. The first dimension "Foundational knowledge and skills" obtained scores above the mean. Knowing the material and equipment, as well as having previous experience in the operating room were the items with the best scores; which reflects that both dimensions of a technical nature are basic and therefore are identified as prior essential theoretical instructions to obtain a clinically relevant competence [15].

The study carried out in Australia with a sample of 345 operating room nurses supports our results, as the authors also reported that experience was a critical factor in ensuring a good level of competence [9]; furthermore, a recently published review insists on the lack of specialized training for nurses in surgical areas and identifies this lack of training as a risk factor associated with certain adverse events; these include intraoperative infections, inappropriate drug administration, or incorrect execution of procedures [16].

Regarding the technical dimension of "Proficiency", the lowest mean value obtained was on the item that evaluates the sufficient amount of knowledge to offer specialized care. The surgical environment is an excessively technocratic and changing context, and having situational awareness is an influential factor in minimizing the risk in adverse situations faced by professionals and favoring their ability to react [17].

The perioperative competence, in addition to including technical competencies, also includes cognitive, affective and psychomotor competencies, focused on comprehensive care based on communication and empathy, both with the patient and with the professional team [2]. These non-technical competencies include the dimension "Professional development", where, specifically, the item "I read current journals and literature related to clinical practice", obtained a low mean value (2.90 ± 1.026), a worrying result since it is the professional's responsibility to have up-to-date knowledge. The same occurs with the dimensions "Leadership" and "Collaboration", with results below those obtained in 2012 by Gillespie et al., [2]. However, the "Empathy" dimension obtained slightly better results and it should be noted here that empathy can be a strength to enhance emotional intelligence as a mechanism that stimulates knowledge and lays the foundations to build stronger teams, improve leadership, the environment and ultimately the quality of care [18, 19].

When we correlated age with the PPCS-R scale, we observe that as age increased, the results improved in the "Knowledge and skills" and "Professional development" dimensions. Both dimensions include the possession of specialized knowledge and its implementation. Regarding the relationship between years worked and the score on the PPCS-R scale, 61.7% had been practicing their profession in the surgical area for more than 10 years, and the results show the highest correlations in items that include possession of specialized knowledge and its application. These results can be based on clinical experience as an indispensable factor and a promoter of training [15, 20].

The trend found in this study relates a greater number of years worked, or in other words the work experience, with the contractual modality. Significant differences are observed between the different contractual models; being the "Permanent" contract model, the one that implies the greatest number of years worked, the one that presents the best results on the PPCS-R scale. In this sense, professionals with a permanent contract have a greater ability to anticipate the situations and needs of a surgical act; they also perceive that they have sufficient knowledge to identify situations of potential or real risk.

Finally, it should be noted that in the surgical field, not only the development of technological competencies should be prioritized, but also competencies related to care and specialized knowledge [21, 22]. The regulated acquisition of these competences, the experience and the continuous training within the clinical field [23, 24] are the tools the professional can count on to promote a culture of safety within the surgical field.

4.1 Limitations

The most important limitation of the present study was related to the appearance of the pandemic caused by SARS-CoV-2. This event made it impossible to continue with data collection, as most of the professionals in the surgical area were relocated to other areas of greater clinical need. Even so, this study can be a starting point to resume data collection and carry it out at a multicenter level. The authors are considering the option of distributing the questionnaire through the Spanish Association of Surgical Nursing (AEEQ).

5. Conclusions

Nurses in surgical areas need to have specific competencies that facilitate the performance of their work and promote quality of care.

The results obtained in the assessment of technical competencies show acceptable values, although these could be improved through training in specific competencies.

Non-technical competencies, such as empathy, are successful; however, the dimension that evaluated leadership scored poorly. A second and third level training would consolidate sufficient knowledge to develop leadership competencies.

Finally, it is observed that with increasing age and increasing number of years worked, the dimensions are better assessed. The same occurs with the type of contractual modality; the "permanent" contractual figure is the one with the best scores. This leads us to conclude that experience is essential to anticipate needs and prevent unwanted adverse events.

Acknowledgements

This study was conducted after obtaining approval from the Clinical Reseach Commission of the Castellón Health Department on March 10th, 2020.

The study did not receive any public or private funding.

The authors thank the HGUCS nursing department for the support received to carry out this study, as well as the interest shown.

Conflict of interest

The authors declare that they have no conflict of interest.

Author details

María Desamparados Bernat Adell[1,2*], María Sánchez Galán[1], Ana Folch Ayora[2], Pablo Salas Molina[2] and Eladio Joaquín Collado Boira[2]

1 General University Hospital of Castellón, Castellón, Spain

2 Nursing Department, Faculty of Health Sciences, Jaume I University, Castellón, Spain

*Address all correspondence to: bernatm@uji.es

References

[1] Organización Colegial de Enfermería. Organización Colegial de Enfermería: Consejo General de Colegios Oficiales de Enfermería de España. Retrieved from: https://www.consejogeneralenfermeria.org/primer-ciclo/grado-en-enfermeria

[2] Gillespie B, Polit D, Hamlin L, Chaboyer W. Developing a model of competence in the operating theatre: Psychometric validation of the Perceived Perioperative Competence Scale-Revised. Int J Nurs Stud. 2012; 49(1): 90-101. Doi: 10.1016/j.ijnurstu.2011.08.001

[3] Ley 44/2003, de 21 de noviembre, de ordenación de las profesiones sanitarias. Boletín oficial del Estado Núm. 280, España, 22 de noviembre de 2003. Retrieved from: https://www.boe.es/buscar/act.php?id=BOE-A-2003-21340

[4] Real Decreto 450/2005, de 22 de abril, sobre especialidades de Enfermería. Boletín Oficial del Estado Núm.108, España, 6 de mayo del 2005, 15480-15486. Retrieved from: https://www.boe.es/diario_boe/txt.php?id=BOE-A-2005-7354

[5] Oltra-Rodríguez E, Rich-Ruiz M, Orts-Cortés M, Sánchez-López D, González-Carrión P. Competencias de investigación en las especialidades de Enfermería. Enferm Clín. 2013; 23(5): 225-230. Doi: 10.1016/j.enfcli.2013.07.006

[6] Vogelsang A, Swenne C, Gustafsson B, Falk-Brynhildsen K. Operating theatre nurse specialist competence to ensure patient safety in the operating theatre: A discursive paper. Nursing Open. 2019; 0(0): 1-8. Doi: 10.1002/nop2.424

[7] Blomberg AC, Lindwall L, Bisholt B. Operating theatre nurses' self-reported clinical competence in perioperative nursing: A mixed method study. Nursing Open. 2019; 6(4):1510-1518. Doi: 10.1002/nop2.352

[8] Blomberg A, Bisholt B, Lindwall L. Responsability for patient care in perioperative practice. Nursing Open. 2018; 5(3): 414-421. Doi: 10.1002/nop2.153

[9] Gillespie B, Chaboyer W, Wallis M, Werder H. Education and Experience Make a Difference: Results of a Predictor Study. AORN Journal. 2011; 94(1): 78-90. Doi: 10.1016/j.aorn.2010.11.037

[10] AORN Position Statement on Perioperative Registered Nurse Circulator Dedicated to Every Patient Undergoing an Operative or Other Invasive Procedure. AORN Journal. 2019; 110(1): 82-85. Doi: 10.1002/aorn.12741

[11] Sillero A, Zabalegui A. Satisfaction of surgical patients with perioperative nursing care in a Spanish tertiary care hospital. SAGE Open Med. 2018; 6(0): 1-9. Doi: 10.1177/2050312118818304

[12] Ingvarsdottir E, Halldorsdottir S. Enhancing patient safety in the operating theatre: from the perspective of experienced operating theatre nurses. Scand J Caring Sci. 2018; 32(2): 951-960. Doi: 10.1111/scs.12532

[13] Ley Orgánica 3/2018, de 5 de diciembre, de Protección de Datos Personales y garantía de los derechos digitales. Boletín Oficial del Estado núm. 294, de 6 de diciembre de 2018, 119788-119857. Madrid: Agencia Estatal Boletín Oficial del Estado. Retrieved from: https://www.boe.es/buscar/doc.php?id=BOE-A-2018-16673

[14] Asociación Médica Mundial. Declaración de Helsinki de la AMM – Principios éticos para las investigaciones médicas en seres humanos. The World Medical Association. 2017. Retrieved

from: https://www.wma.net/es/policies-post/declaracion-de-helsinki-de-la-amm-principios-eticos-para-las-investigaciones-medicas-en-seres-humanos/

[15] Stobinski JX. Perioperative Nursing Competency. AORN Journal. 2008; 88(3), 417-436. Doi: 10.1016/j.aorn.2008.05.001

[16] Beitz JM. Addressing the Perioperative Nursing Shortage Through Education: A Perioperative Imperative. AORN Journal. 2019; 110(4): 403-414. Doi: 10.1002/aorn.12805

[17] Cronenwett L, Sherwood G, Barnsteiner J, Disch J, Johnson J, Mitchell P, Sullivan D, Warren J. Initial psychometric evaluation of the nursing quality and safety self-inventory. J Nurs Educ. 2007; 52(5): 269-274. Doi: 10.1016/j.outlook.2007.02.006

[18] Sandelin A, Gustafsson BÅ. Operating theatre nurses' experiences of teamwork for safe surgery. Nordic J Nurs Res. 2015; 35(3): 179-185. Doi: 10.1177/0107408315591337

[19] Beydler KW. The rol of Emotional Intelligence in Perioperative Nursing and Leadership: Developing Skills for Improved Performance. AORN Journal. 2017; 106(4): 317-323. Doi: 10.1016/j.aorn.2017.08.002

[20] Manchester J, Palma S, Karasin M. Closing the gap: A regional partnership model for perioperative nursing. J Contin Educ Nurs. 2019; 50(8): 363-366. Doi: 10.3928/00220124-20190717-07

[21] Smith J, Palesy D. Technology stress in perioperative nursing: An ongoing concern. Journal of Perioperative Nursing. 2018; 31(2):24-28. Doi: 10.26550/2209-1092.1028

[22] Van Wicklin AhA, Leveling ME, Stobinski JX. What Is the Perceived Value of Certification Among Registered Nurses? A Systematic Review J Nurs Scholars. 2020; 52(5): 536-543. Doi: 10.1111/jnu.12579

[23] Lozito M, Whiteman K, Swanson-Biearman B, Barkhymer M, Stephens K. Goog Catch Campaign: Improving the Perioperative Culture of Safety. AORN Journal. 2018; 107(6): 705-714. Doi: 10.1002/aorn.12148

[24] Habahbeh AA, Alkhalaileh MA. Effect of an educational programme on the attitudes towards patient safety of operation room nurses. Br J Nurs. 2020; 29(4): 222-228. Doi: 10.12968/bjon.2020.29.4.222

Chapter 9

The Use of Virtual Reality Simulations in Nursing Education, and Patient Safety

Sule Biyik Bayram and Nurcan Caliskan

Abstract

Nursing education puts theory into practice. Patient safety is indispensable in nursing education. During clinical practice, nursing students make medication errors and have difficulty deciding on what interventions to perform in unusual situations and communicating with patients or other healthcare professionals. All these problems put patient safety at risk. However, "First, do no harm" is a fundamental human right and an ethical principle, which nurses should always consider when they perform interventions. Nursing students can help develop a culture of patient safety through experience in line with their knowledge, skills, and affective goals. Clinical settings can be equipped with real-life laboratories, mannequins, etc. Virtual reality simulations show nursing students what it is like to be in a real-world clinical setting and what problems and risks they may encounter there, and thus, helps them develop skills, build confidence, and prepare for clinical practice. This section addressed the effect of virtual reality simulations on skill development and patient safety in nursing education.

Keywords: nursing education, patient safety, psychomotor skills, simulation, virtual reality

1. Introduction

Nursing education integrates theory and practice to help students develop cognitive, intellectual, affective (attitudes and beliefs), and psychomotor skills and prepare for professional life [1]. Errors in real clinical settings threaten patient safety. Therefore, nursing students should perform primary nursing interventions over and over in laboratories and develop basic psychomotor skills before they enter clinical practice. Simulations replicate real-world situations in which nursing students can gain clinical experience without putting patients at risk [1–3]. Simulations provide effective learning environments where nursing students can gain experience and develop collaboration, management, critical thinking, communication, clinical decision-making, and problem-solving skills without harming patients, and boost their confidence and readiness for real clinical practice [2, 4–6]. Virtual reality (VR), which is a type of simulation, consists of state-of-the-art equipment and augmented-reality interventions. The more similar the simulation is to the real clinical setting, the more motivated and better the students are at developing skills. VR simulations provide nursing students with the opportunity to perform high-risk and high-cost interventions on virtual patients and gain experience without jeopardizing the safety of real patients [7, 8].

1.1 Psychomotor skills and simulations

Psychomotor skills are coordinated muscle movements governed by conscious mental processes to complete certain tasks [9]. Students develop psychomotor skills by putting theory into practice in lab settings. Instructors first demonstrate the skills and then allow students to put them into practice by themselves and give them feedback on their performance until they become competent [10]. In lab settings, students analyze theoretical knowledge, learn to make observations, and establish a relationship between theory and practice, put their critical thinking and problem-solving skills into practice, and build up confidence [11, 12]. This training teaches them how to perform interventions before clinical practice without risking patient safety [3, 5]. Nursing students without psychomotor skills are more likely to feel insecure and inadequate and make medical errors in clinical practice than those with psychomotor skills [5]. To overcome those problems, it is necessary to help nursing students acquire knowledge and develop skills and put the theoretical knowledge of safe care into practice. Educational technologies are recommended to achieve that goal [13–15]. The students of Generation Z are particularly interested in technology and can easily access information via their personal devices. Therefore, simulations that appeal to the new generation of students have become widespread [5].

Simulations are a safe way for students to perform activities in environments that replicate actual or potential situations. It is effective and engaging because it helps students learn how to use equipment and develop problem-solving and decision-making skills before they step into real clinical settings where training is hard, dangerous, and costly. Simulations are used for pilot and astronaut training and medical education (e.g., cadaver) [16]. Simulations allow nursing students to practice whenever they want without jeopardizing patient safety [17, 18].

1.2 Types of simulations

Two types of simulations are used in nursing education; high-fidelity and low-fidelity. Low-fidelity simulations are three-dimensional organ models, human cadavers, animal models, and simulated and standardized patients. Three-dimensional organ models are anatomical models used to teach students about cardiac functions and how to insert a peripheral IV catheter and perform spinal anesthesia, first aid for injuries, and a breast examination. Simulated and standardized patients are used to help students develop communication skills and to teach them how to take a medical history and perform physical examinations [19]. High-fidelity simulations are image-based, realistic, and interactive patient simulations, VR, and haptic systems. Image-based simulations are computerized image-and video-based simulations that help students learn and develop critical thinking and decision-making skills by themselves [20]. Realistic and interventional simulations, also known as partial task trainers, imitate body parts to teach students particular skills. Some of the realistic and interventional simulations are models for intravascular and foley catheterization, and stitching, and eye and ear as well as ultrasound, clinical cardiology (auscultation), and invasive cardiology (catheterization) simulations. High-tech interactive simulations are computerized virtual patients replicating human anatomy and physiology. Such simulations can breathe, talk, and move their eyes, and have a pulse and heart rate [21]. VR and haptic systems are three-dimensional simulations that feel real and communicate with participants through computers [22]. Haptic systems are used to tutor students on laparoscopic and endoscopic interventions and to evaluate surgical skills [23].

1.3 Virtual reality

Virtual reality is a computer-generated 3-D simulation that delivers a wide range of sensory information to the user to allow them to interact with objects in a virtual environment and make them feel like they are physically there [15, 24]. VR can be used to help nursing students develop skills in virtual hospital settings.

Interactivity is a key feature of VR, making it more effective than video demonstration. In VR simulations, users wear 3-D glasses and data suits and interact with one another haptically or via a keyboard and a mouse [24–28]. Second Life, Quest Atlantis, Active Worlds, Wonderland, World of Warcraft, and Opensim are 3D/VR platforms, with Second Life being the most popular one [15].

Virtual reality simulations provide students with the opportunity to put interventions into practice on models to overcome problems they may encounter in real clinics [29]. For example, VR can be used to teach nursing students tracheostomy care or urinary catheterization [17, 29]. In this way, they can develop nursing skills on virtual patients and perform interventions smoothly and confidently in real clinics without running the risk of harming real patients [15].

There are two types of VR technologies; immersive and non-immersive. Immersive means "the state of being surrounded, engrossed, and absorbed, the state of being three-dimensional," as well as "plunging into something, and disassociating from reality and entering a virtual world [30]. Immersive VR provides experiences where the user wears a headset and motion-sensing gloves and loses all sense of the real world in a place no bigger than a room. Non-immersive VR is a computer-generated not-fully interactive 3D environment in which the user uses a keyboard, mouse, joystick, and haptic display to control and navigate [31].

1.4 What is virtual reality, and where is it used?

Virtual reality was first used in video games, followed by education, culture, arts, tourism, e-commerce, manufacturing, military and airline, construction, and production [22]. Three-dimensional virtual worlds in education make students more motivated to access information and use it in learning and help them adopt lifelong learning and develop collaboration skills [32]. Virtual reality also allows students to immerse themselves in virtual worlds that replicate the real world and use the materials there and interact with them. It appeals to all senses and promotes effective learning and learning retention. In the field of education, VR was first used in military, flight, and astronaut training [30]. Packy and Marlon was an educational video game developed in 1995 in Japan to teach self-care behavior to children with diabetes [33].

1.5 The use of virtual reality simulations in nursing education

Virtual reality in the field of medical education is defined as a type of computer-based 3D simulation that makes users feel like they are in clinical settings where they can practice skills without putting patients at risk [15]. VR used in physical therapy, and medical and nursing education [15, 17, 34–37] allows students to practice as often as they want and see their own mistakes in safe lab settings [38]. Therefore, such simulations with active engagement improve learning retention and enable participants to learn interactively and analyze problems [39]. VR serves as a bridge between theory and practice in nursing education [40]. Research shows that VR makes learning fun and active participation possible through feedback and helps nursing students acquire knowledge and develop skills and makes them more motivated and confident [41–44].

Nehring and Lashley [45] mentioned that Phillips [46] was the first to use VR in nursing. Afterward, Merril and Barker [47] developed a prototype for intravenous (IV) catheterization, and then, Skiba [48] used Internet-based interactive virtual environments [45]. The first example of VR in nursing is the CathSim Intravenous Training System (CathSim ITS) developed in 1998. Research shows that CathSim ITS makes participants more motivated and confident and results in a reduction in intervention-related pain, the incidence of hematoma formation, and the number of interventions [49–51]. Students with low anxiety and advanced skills are more likely to perform initiatives quickly and safely. Multiple interventions increase potential risks and jeopardize patient safety.

1.6 Advantages and disadvantages of virtual reality

Virtual reality simulations boost students' concentration, engagement, confidence, motivation, and creativity, and allow them to put theory into practice and learn at their own pace [45]. It also provides them with the opportunity to practice whenever and how often they want in safe and realistic environments without fear of making mistakes and harming patients [52]. Students participating in VR simulations are more likely to become comfortable, confident, and successful in real clinical settings because they learn in an applied format [17, 29]. They can also practice dangerous, costly, and complex interventions that they are less likely to encounter in real clinics [22]. However, VR simulations require interdisciplinary collaboration, and time and money to design scenarios and to train instructors [28]. Besides, prolonged VR use causes dizziness, headaches, and pain when moving the eyes [53].

1.7 Impact of virtual reality simulations on patient safety

Patient safety is about eliminating preventable medical errors that cause harm to patients [54]. High-quality nursing education is a precondition of patient safety. Simulations, in general, and VR, in particular, improve the quality of nursing education and enables students to put theory into practice and develop skills and positive attitudes [15]. Those students are more likely to consider patient safety when performing clinical interventions [55].

Research shows that students who have developed fundamental nursing skills in virtual environments are likely to feel more comfortable and confident and minimize the harm that may result from interventions in real clinical settings [9, 10]. For example, Tag Team Patient Safety Simulation (TTPSS) enhanced nursing students' knowledge and skills and enabled them to provide safe care [56]. VR simulation scenarios should emphasize the principles of patient safety to teach students how to provide safe care in clinics. The Joint Commission International outlines six principles of patient safety [57, 58]. The next section discusses the contribution of VR simulations to nursing education with reference to those principles.

2. Identifying patients correctly

Patient identity should be confirmed before all fundamental nursing interventions. The patient should have at least two of the four identifiers (name, surname, protocol number, and date of birth) as evidence for identification [59]. Skill tests

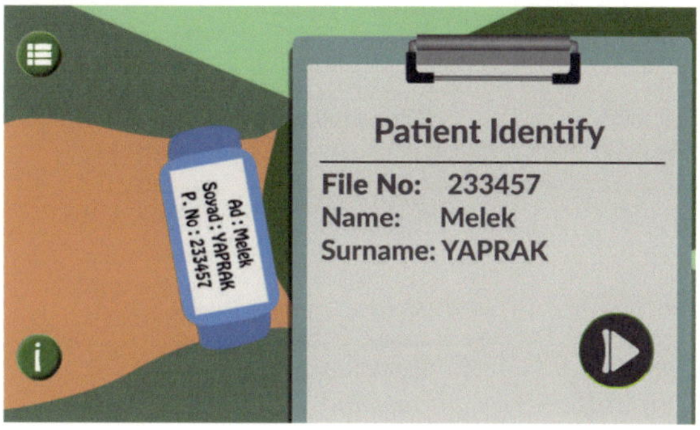

Figure 1.
Patient identify.

and lists in nursing education emphasize the importance of patient identification. Henneman et al. [60] emphasized in his simulation study that verification of patient identity before drug administration is important in ensuring patient safety.
In a VR simulation scenario on tracheostomy care, an avatar nurse verified the identity of a virtual patient from her wristband and explained to her the medical procedure to be carried out [61]. The scenario taught the participants how to identify patients correctly. It also highlighted the significance of patient identification as an essential stage of clinical interventions by not allowing the participants who failed to verify the patient's identity to move on to the next stage. Therefore, such scenarios are an effective method for teaching nursing students how to identify patients correctly.

In the studies, the first step in the teaching of skill is the patient character verification process [43, 62, 63]. In a thesis study conducted by Biyik Bayram [62], one of the process steps in the simulation scenario is the patient verification step. Performing the student patient verification process in the VR game will enable him to focus on the same step in the clinic (**Figure 1**) [62]. Koivisto et al. [43], in their study with 166 nursing students, stated that students working with a simulation scenario were able to identify the descriptive characteristics of the patient and plan appropriate nursing interventions. Shibuy et al. [63] in his study with 36 nursing students, it is expected that the student will verify the patient identity in the first step in the 24-item tracheostomy aspiration skill. As seen in the studies, nursing skills practices start with the verification step of the patient identity and the student must ensure the competence in simulation practice to fulfill this task in clinical practice (**Table 1**) [63].

3. Improving effective communication

All healthcare professionals should have effective communication skills to ensure patient safety. Research shows that a lack of or poor communication or miscommunication among patients, nurses, and other healthcare professionals puts patient safety at risk [56, 72]. A lack of communication leads to missing patient data and poor planning, which may result in misdiagnosis and inappropriate treatment [72]. High-fidelity simulations help healthcare professionals develop communication skills. Low-fidelity partial body manikins cannot give feedback, but high-fidelity Simman and virtual patients can speak [64]. VR simulations that can talk enable students to cooperate and make accurate and rapid clinical decisions [73]. Similarly, communicating with virtual patients improve students' communication skills (**Table 1**) [56, 64–66]. VR can be used to teach students how to take patient history,

Patient safety principles	Author/year	Design	Method	Conclusion
1. Identify patient correctly	Shibuya et al./2019 [63]	Three groups	Virtual Reality (VR group) Traditional demonstration (TR group) No intervention (NO group):	The checklist of tracheostomy suctioning skills (Identify patient using name)
	Biyik Bayram/2017 [62]	Randomized controlled	Game Based Virtual Reality (experimental group) Traditional method (control group)	The checklist of tracheostomy care skills (Identify patient using wristband)
	Koivisto et al./2016 [43]	Descriptive study	CareMe® Virtual Reality Game	It has been stated that simulation is effective patient identification.
	Henneman et al./2010 [60]	Retrospective study	Two simulation scenarios	It has been determined that the nursing process game increases students' concentration and experience.
2. Improving effective communication	Fay-Hiller et al./2012 [55]	Review	High-fidelity simulations	Health team communication.
	Guise et al./2012 [65]	Review	High-fidelity simulations	Simulation help healthcare professionals develop communication skills.
	Foronda et al./2016 [65]	Descriptive and mix method	Virtual reality simulation	Strengthens team communication
	Liu et al./2018 [66]	Pilot study	Virtual patients	Virtual patient improves students' communication skills
3. Improving the safety of high-alert medications	Gu et al./2017 [67]	Randomized controlled	Virtual reality simulations	It was stated that the IV drug infusion skills of the students increased. Prevents medication administration errors.
	Lutckar-Flude et al./2012 [68]	Experimental study	The laboratory study (control group) Virtual learning module (experimental group)	It was stated that the students' self-confidence increased.
	Dubovi et al./2017 [69]	Quasi--experimental study (pre-post test)	Virtual Reality Simulation	Learned well about drug management
	Vidal et al./2013 [49]	Quasi--experimental study	Intravenous Virtual Reality Simulation	Intravenous catheter interventions more successfully

Patient safety principles	Author/year	Design	Method	Conclusion
4. Ensuring correct site	Kruglikova et al./2010 [70]	Experimental study	The Accu Touch endoscopy simulator	Virtual Reality colonoscopy simulation performed it more accurately, safely, and quickly.
	Weideman and Culleiton/2014 [71]	Review	Virtual patient	Virtual patient improved students' obstetrics skills.

Table 1.
The studies of contribution of virtual reality simulations on 1,2,3 and 4 patient safety principles.

welcome patients to the clinic, implement the protocol/procedure for discharge, and communicate with other healthcare professionals.

4. Improving the safety of high-alert medications

Nurses frequently administer medications based on the six rights: the right drug, the right patient, the right dose, the right route, the right time, and the right documentation. Nurses who do not comply with those principles or do not know how to administer drugs or have never practiced on a model are more likely to put patient safety at risk [74]. VR simulations give students feedback and help them learn by doing interactively [67]. VR simulations on intravenous drug infusion [67, 68] and administration [70] help students improve the ability to administer medications safely. Dubovi et al. [69] found that nursing students who participated in a VR simulation learned well about drug management. Gu et al. [67] also reported that a VR simulation helped nursing students acquire knowledge on the fundamental principles of asepsis, urinary catheterization, and drug management. Luctkar-Flude et al. [68] found that a VR simulation improved nursing students' IV drug infusion skills. VR simulations are also used to teach nursing students how to notice possible complications after drug administration. For example, Vidal et al. [49] determined that nursing students performed IV interventions more successfully on fewer trials, inflicted less pain on patients, and observed lower incidence of hematoma formation after they participated in a VR simulation (**Table 1**). This result suggests that nursing students participating in VR simulations comply with the six rights of drug administration and intervention steps, and thus, prevent complications, resulting in improved patient compliance and shortened length of hospital stay.

5. Ensuring correct-site, correct-procedure, correct-patient surgery

Surgical errors are among the most common errors that jeopardize patient safety. Virtual patients can be used to inform students on patient safety based on the Surgical Safety Checklist. Students can practice filling out the name and location of the surgery and receiving informed consent before surgery. In this way, they can see their shortcomings and evaluate patient outcomes and learn better through experience [53]. Medical students can manage or perform surgeries on virtual patients that replicate human anatomy and cope with complications [40]. Nurses practicing colonoscopy [70] and obstetric [68] interventions on virtual patients are likely to have better skills and make fewer errors. Kruglikova et al. [70] found that nurses participating in a VR colonoscopy simulation performed it more accurately, safely, and quickly. Weideman and Culleiton [71]. reported that practicing obstetrics on a virtual patient improved students' skill (**Table 1**). This result shows that virtual patients can be used to help surgical nursing students see their shortcomings and patient outcomes and develop skills.

6. Reducing the risk of health care-associated infections

Infections are the most common cause of death in hospitals. Hand and skin hygiene before each intervention breaks the chain of infection [75]. VR simulations can be used to help nurses develop positive attitudes towards hygiene, resulting in a reduction in the rate of infections. Hand washing is the most effective way to prevent the spread of infections. Nakamura et al. [76] found that simulation scenarios raised students' awareness of hand hygiene and reduced the incidence of catheter-infection. VR simulations improve students' knowledge and skills on decontamination [44, 77] and urinary [4, 17] and intravenous catheterization [10, 34, 78, 79], port catheter injection [35], tracheostomy aspiration [80] and care [29] and nasogastric (NG) tube insertion (**Table 2**) [50, 83]. Failure to comply with asepsis rules in such invasive procedures may cause the spread of infections. Besides, students rarely find themselves in situations where they have to perform those procedures in clinics. They should, nevertheless, practice them in VR simulations so that they would not have anxiety and difficulties in case they have to perform them in clinics [15]. This enables them to put their knowledge and skills into practice more efficiently, resulting in higher-quality care and reduced rates of infections and complications.

In the experimental study conducted by Smith and Hamilton [44] with 20 nursing students, it was stated that computer-based VR application increased urinary catheter skills. In the study conducted by Kardong-Edgren et al. [4] with 31 nursing students, it was stated that haptic VR application increased urinary catheterization skills. These studies highlight the asepsis conditions that the student must comply with in the urinary catheterization procedure. It is aimed that the student fulfills the requirements of asepsis while performing this procedure on the patient. Butt et al. [17] performed urinary catheterization skills with 20 nursing students in a VR environment with a device and gloves they wore on their heads. In a study conducted by Farra et al. [77] with 106 nursing students, it was stated that students' decontamination skills increased. Thus, attention was paid to the prevention of infections. Tsai et al. [34] stated that the frequency of errors of students decreased in the intravenous catheter application they performed in virtual environment with 10 students. In the study conducted by Jung et al. [78], it was stated that the success of the group working with intravenous catheter application and arm model was higher than the others. Tsai et al. [35] increased the knowledge level of port catheter injection of 77 nurses using VR application. Noyudom et al. [80] increased tracheostomy aspiration skills of 35 nursing students working in a virtual environment.

Biyik Bayram and Caliskan [29] stated that 86 nursing students increased tracheostomy aspiration skills with the use of VR. In the study conducted by Chiang et al. [50] with 79 students, it was stated that NG tube insertion application skills increased. NG tube insertion skill is a procedure that must be complied with medical asepsis conditions. Thus, the student understands the distinction between medical and surgical asepsis rules. Similarly, VRapplications are designed to improve NG tube insertion skills in the design study by Choi and his friends.

Patient safety principles	Author/Year	Design	Method	Conclusion
5. Reducing the risk of infections	Smith and Hamilton/2015 [44]	Experimental study	Computer-based virtual reality	The urinary catheterization skills have increased.
	Farra et al./2015 [77]	Quasi--experimental	Virtual reality	The decontamination skills of the students increased.
	Kardong-Edgren et al./2019 [4]	Pilot study	Haptik and virtual reality	Virtual reality is fun and effective in teaching.
	Butt et al./2018 [17]	Pilot study	İmmersive virtual reality	Students' level of knowledge is increased
	Tsai et al./2008 [34]	Pilot study	Virtual reality	Intravenous catheter application skill was advanced.
	Jung et al./2012 [78]	Experimental study	Arm model (A group) Virtual reality (B group) Virtual reality and arm model (C group)	C group was successful compared to other groups.
	Engum et al./2003 [79]	Randomized controlled (Pre-post test)	Arm model (control group) Virtual reality (experimental group)	There was an increase in the intravenous catheter application knowledge scores of the students who used the virtual reality method.
	Tsai et al./2008 [35]	Experimental study (Pre-post test)	Traditional (control group) Virtual reality (experimental group)	Port catheter injection knowledge and skill increased.
	Noyudom et al./2011 [80]	Experimental (Pre-post test)	Virtual Reality	Tracheostomy suctioning knowledge and skill increased.
	Biyik Bayram and Caliskan/2019 [29]	Randomized controlled	Traditional (control group) Virtual reality (experimental group)	Tracheostomy care knowledge and skill increased.
	Chiang et al./2017 [50]	Quasi--experimental	Traditional (control group) Virtual reality (experimental group)	NG tube insertion skill increased.
	Choi et al./2015 [78]	Pilot study	Virtual reality	Thought to guide nurses.
6. Reducing the risk of patient falls	Bursiek et al./2020 [81]	Pilot study	Virtual scenario	Patient falls decreased.
	DeBourg and Prion/2011 [82]	Quasi-experimental study (per-post test)	Simulation	Simulation ensuring a culture of patient safety and preventing falls.

Table 2.
The studies of contribution of virtual reality simulations on 5 and 6 patient safety principles.

7. Reducing the risk of patient harm resulting from falls

Nurses are responsible for providing safe care, which is an indicator of the quality of care [70]. Making sure the bed brakes are locked and raising the bed rails are preventive measures against accidental falls. Therefore, VR simulations are used to teach them. Biyik Bayram and Caliskan [61] used a tracheostomy care scenario in which the student was supposed to lower the bed rails before the intervention and raise them back after the intervention, and if the student skipped the step, she failed to complete it. Such simulations teach students what kind of preventive measures to take against falls. Bursiek et al. [81] reported a decrease in patient falls in clinics with nurses working in virtual scenarios. It was also emphasized that teamwork is effective in preventing patient falls [81]. DeBourg et al. [82] stated that simulation studies were effective in providing patient safety culture of 285 students and preventing falls (**Table 2**). VR simulations have scenarios in which students can keep practicing preventive measures against falls. In this way, they know what to do when they encounter such situations in real clinics. Students should put virtual patients in VR simulations at risk so that they will not jeopardize the safety of real patients because the former can afford the risk, but the latter cannot.

8. Conclusions

Nursing education is an applied type of education. Therefore, students must perform both lab and clinical practice. However, students may put patients at risk because they are inexperienced. Nurses are responsible for establishing a culture of patient safety and protecting patients. Nursing students should participate in activities and lab interventions to become aware of patient safety. Nursing students who do not have much opportunity to participate in lab activities can be provided with VR simulations. Research shows that VR simulations help students gain knowledge and develop collaboration and critical thinking skills, and recognize rare clinical situations, and communicate effectively with patients. Nursing students with those skills can provide safe care, administer medications correctly, and notice changes in their patients. In conclusion, students who participate in VR simulations can provide patient safety in real clinics.

Conflict of interest

No conflict of interest has been declared by the authors.

Glossary of abbreviations

VR	Virtual Reality
IV	Intravenous
NG	Nasogastric
TTPSS	Tag Team Patient Safety Simulation

Author details

Sule Biyik Bayram[1*] and Nurcan Caliskan[2]

1 Department of Nursing, Faculty of Health Sciences, Karadeniz Technical University, Trabzon, Turkey

2 Department of Nursing, Faculty of Health Sciences, Gazi University, Ankara, Turkey

*Address all correspondence to: sulebiyik@gmail.com

References

[1] Oermann MH, Gaberson KB. Evaluation and Testing In Nursing Education. 4th ed. New York; Springer Publishing Company; 2014. 12-305p.

[2] Cant RP, Cooper SJ. Simulation based learning in nurse education: systematic review. Journal of Advanced Nursing. 2010;**66**(1):3-15. DOI: 10.1111/j.1365-2648.2009.05240.x

[3] Silveira MDS, Cogo ALP. The contributions of digital technologies in the teaching of nursing skills: an integrative review. Revista gaucha de enfermagem. 2017;38(2). DOI: 10.1590/1983-1447.2017.02.66204

[4] Kardong-Edgren S, Breitkreuz K, Werb M, Foreman S, Ellertson A. Evaluating the usability of a second-generation virtual reality game for refreshing sterile urinary catheterization skills. Nurse educator. 2019;**44**(3):137-141. DOI: 10.1097/NNE.0000000000000570

[5] Terzioğlu F, Kapucu S, Özdemir L, Boztepe H, Duygulu S, Tuna Z, et al. Nursing students' opinions about simulation method. Hacettepe University Nursing Faculty Journal. 2012;**19**(1):16-23 (in Turkish)

[6] Khalaila R. Simulation in nursing education: an evaluation of students' out comes at their first clinical practice combined with simulations. Nurse Education Today. 2014;**34**(2):252-258. DOI: 10.1016/j.nedt.2013.08.015

[7] Raman S, Labrague LJ, Arulappan J, Natarajan J, Amirtharaj A, Jacob D. Traditional clinical training combined with high-fidelity simulation-based activities improves clinical competency and knowledge among nursing students on a maternity nursing course. In Nursing Forum. 2019;**54**(3):434-440. DOI: 10.1111/nuf.12351

[8] Fealy S, Jones D, Hutton A, Graham K, McNeill L, Sweet L, et al. The integration of immersive virtual reality in tertiary nursing and midwifery education: A scoping review. Nurse Education Today. 2019;**79**:14-19. DOI: 10.1016/j.nedt.2019.05.002

[9] Morgan R. Using clinical skills laboratories to promote theory–practice integration during first practice placement: an Irish perspective. Journal of Clinical Nursing. 2006;**15**(2):155-161. DOI: 10.1111/j.1365-2702.2006.01237.x

[10] Baillie L, Curzio J. A survey of first year student nurses' experiences of learning blood pressure measurement. Nurse Education in Practice. 2009;**9**:61-71. DOI: 10.1016/j.nepr.2008.05.003

[11] Mete S, Uysal N. Implementatıon of an Education Model for Nursing Skills Development Dokuz Eylül University High School Nursing E-journal. 2009;2(3), 115-123. http://hdl.handle.net/20.500.12397/4532 (in Turkish).

[12] Eker F, Açıkgöz F, Karaca A. Occupational Skill Training through the Eyes of Nursing Students. Dokuz Eylül University High School Nursing E-journal. 2014;7(4):291-294 http://www.deuhyoedergi.org/index.php/DEUHYOED/article/view/123/365 (in Turkish)

[13] Kelly M, Lyng C, McGrath M, Cannon G. A multi-method study to determine the effectiveness of, and student attitudes to, online instructional videos for teaching clinical nursing skills. Nurse Education Today. 2009;**29**(3):292-300. DOI: 10.1016/j.nedt.2008.09.004

[14] Aleman JLF, De Gea JMC, Mondejar JJR. Effects of competitive computer-assisted learning versus conventional teaching methods on the acquisition and retention of knowledge

in medical surgical nursing students. Nurse Education Today. 2011;**31**(8):866-871. DOI: 10.1016/j.nedt.2010.12.026

[15] Jenson CE, Forsythm DM. Virtual reality simulation: using three-dimensional technology to teach nursing students. Computers Informatics Nursing. 2012;**30**(6):312-318. DOI: 10.1097/NXN.0b013e31824af6ae

[16] Tan Ş. Öğretim Ilke ve Yöntemleri. 13rd ed. Ankara: Pegem Akademi; 2016. pp. 2-307 (in Turkish)

[17] Butt AL, Kardong-Edgren S, Ellertson A. Using game-based virtual reality with haptics for skill acquisition. Clinical Simulation Nursing. 2018;**16**:25-32. DOI: 10.1016/j.ecns.2017.09.010

[18] Şendir M, Doğan P. Hemşirelik eğitiminde simülasyonun kullanımı: Sistematik inceleme. Florence Nightingale Nursing Journal. 2015;**23**(1):49-56 (in Turkish)

[19] Ziv A, Small SD, Wolpe PR. Patient safety and simulation-based medical education. Medical Teacher. 2000;**22**(5):489-495. DOI: 10.1080/01421590050110777

[20] Lane JL, Slavin S, Ziv A. Simulation in medical education: A review. Simulation & Gaming. 2001;**32**(3):297-314. DOI: 10.1177/104687810103200302

[21] Mıdık Ö, Kartal M. Simulation-based medical education. Marmara Medical Journal. 2010;**23**(3):389-399 http://hdl.handle.net/11424/1925

[22] Bayraktar E, Kaleli F. Virtual reality on commercial applications Akademik Bilişim 2007. 1-6.

[23] Çoban S. Uzaktan ve teknoloji destekli eğitimin gelişimi. 2012. Available from: http://inet-tr.org.tr/inetconf17/bildiri/26.pdf. [Accessed: 2020-06-30]

[24] Bulu ST, İşler V. Second life ODTÜ kampüsü. Akademik Bilişim Kongresi'nde sunulan bildiri. İnönü Üniversitesi, Malatya: Kasım, 15, 2011.

[25] Aydın ED. Üç boyutlu sanal gerçeklik ortamında mimari mekan temsilinin geliştirilmesi: temel anlam ve yan anlam yaratma, [thesis]. Fen Bilimleri Enstitüsü, İstanbul: Yıldız Teknik Üniversitesi; 2012

[26] Kaufman D, Sauve L. Educational gameplay and simulation environments: case studies and lessons learned: Case studies and lessons learned. New York: Information Science Reference; 2010. pp. 231-250p

[27] Sherman WR, Craig AB. Understanding virtual reality: Interface, application, and design. USA: Elsevier. 2003. 24-37p.

[28] Kayabaşı Y. Sanal gerçeklik ve egitim amaçlı kullanılması. The Turkish Online Journal of Educational Technology. 2005;**4**(3):151-166 http://www.tojet.net/volumes/v4i3.pdf#page=151

[29] Biyik Bayram S, Caliskan N. Effect of a game-based virtual reality phone application on tracheostomy care education for nursing students: a randomised controlled trial. Nurse Education Today. 2019;**79**:25-31. DOI: 10.1016/j.nedt.2019.05.010

[30] Tepe T, Kaleci D, Tüzün H. Eğitim teknolojilerinde yeni eğilimler: sanal gerçeklik uygulamaları. Paper presented at the 10th International Computer and Instructional Technologies Symposium. 2016. Rize, Türkiye.

[31] Lee EAL, Wong KW. A review of using virtual reality for learning. Heidelberg: Springer; 2008

[32] Erbaş Ç, Demirer V. Eğitimde sanal ve artırılmış gerçeklik uygulamaları. Online Books: Eğitim Teknolojileri Okumaları; 2015. pp. 131-148p

[33] Lupton D. Health promotion in the digital era: a critical commentary. Health promotion international. 2014;**30**(1):174-183. DOI: 10.1093/heapro/dau091

[34] Tsai WW, Fung CP, Tsai SL, Jeng MC, Doong JL. The assessment of stability and reliability of a virtual reality-based intravenous injection simulator. Computers Informatics Nursing. 2008;**26**(4):221-226. DOI: 10.1097/01.NCN.0000304804.46369.5a

[35] Tsai SL, Chai SK, Hsieh LF, Lin S, Taur FM, Sung WH, et al. The use of virtual reality computer simulation in learning Port-A cath injection. Advances in Health Sciences Education. 2008;**13**(1):71-87. DOI: 10.1007/s10459-006-9025-3

[36] Loukas C, Nikiteas N, Kanakis M, Moutsatsos A, Leandros E, Georgiou E. A virtual reality simulation curriculum for intravenous cannulation training. Academic Emergency Medicine. 2010;**17**(10):1142-1145. DOI: 10.1111/j.1553-2712.2010.00876.x

[37] Shin JH, Park SB, Jang SH. Effects of game-based virtual reality on health-related quality of life in chronic stroke patients: A randomized, controlled study. Computers in Biology and Medicine. 2015;**63**:92-98. DOI: 10.1016/j.compbiomed.2015.03.011

[38] Boz Yüksekdağ B. Hemşirelik eğitiminde bilgisayar teknolojisinin kullanımı. Açıköğretim Uygulamaları ve Araştırmaları Dergisi. 2015;**1**(1):103-118 (in Turkish)

[39] Huang HM, Rauch U, Liaw SS. Investigating learners'attitudes toward virtual reality learning environments: Based on a constructivist approach. Computers & Education. 2010;**55**(3):1171-1182. DOI: 10.1016/j.compedu.2010.05.014

[40] Simpson RL. The virtual reality revolution: Technology changes nursing education. Nursing Management. 2002;**33**(9):14-15 http://www.nursingmanagement.com

[41] Chia P. Using a virtual game to enhance simulation based learning in nursing education. Singapore Nursing Journal. 2013;**40**(3):21-26

[42] Lancaster RJ. Serious game simulation as a teaching strategy in pharmacology. Clinical Simulation in Nursing. 2014;**10**(3):129-137. DOI: 10.1016/j.ecns.2013.10.005

[43] Koivisto JM, Niemi H, Multisilta J, Eriksson E. Nursing students' experiential learning processes using an online 3D simulation game. Education and Information Technologies. 2015:1-16. DOI: 10.1007/s10639-015-9453-x

[44] Smith PC, Hamilton BK. The effects of virtual reality simulation as a teaching strategy for skills preparation ın nursing students. Clinical Simulation in Nursing. 2015;**1**(11):52-58. DOI: 10.1016/j.ecns.2014.10.001

[45] Nehring WM, Lashley FR. Nursing simulation: A review of the past 40 years. Simulation & Gaming. 2009;**40**(4):528-552. DOI: 10.1177/1046878109332282

[46] Phillips JR. Virtual reality: A new vista for nurse researchers? *Nursing Science Quarterly*. 1993;*6*(1):5-7

[47] Merril GL, Barker VL. Virtual reality debuts in the teaching laboratory in nursing. *Nurse Educator?* 1996;*19*:182-187

[48] Skiba D. Nursing education 2.0: Second life. *Nursing Education Perspectives*. 2007;*28*:156-157

[49] Vidal VL, Ohaeri BM, John P, Helen D. Virtual reality and the traditional method for phlebotomy training among college of nursing

students in Kuwait: implications for nursing education and practice. Journal of Infusion Nursing. 2013;**36**(5):349-355. DOI: 10.1097/NAN.0b013e318243172f

[50] Chiang VCL, Choi TKS, Ching SSY, Leung, KLK. Evaluation of a virtual reality based interactive simulator with haptic feedback for learning NGT placement. Journal of Problem-Based Learning. 2017; 4(1), 25-34. DOI: 10.24313/jpbl.2017.4.1.25

[51] Jamison RJ, Hovancsek MT, Clochesy JM. A pilot study assessing simulation using two simulation methods for teaching intravenous cannulation. Clinical Simulation in Nursing. 2006;**2**(1):9-12. DOI: 10.1016/j.ecns.2009.05.007

[52] Çavaş B, Çavaş PH, Can BT. Eğitimde sanal gerçeklik. TOJET: The Turkish Online Journal of Educational Technology. 2004;**3**(4):110-116

[53] Aslan R. Uluslararası rekabette yeni imkanlar: sanal gerçeklik, artırılmış gerçeklik ve hologram. Ayrıntı Dergisi. 2017;**5**(49):21-26

[54] National Patient Safety Foundation. Patient safety. 2016. Available from: http://www.npsf.org/?page=dictionarynz [Accessed: 2020-06-30]

[55] Fay-Hillier TM, Regan RV, Gallagher GM. Communication and patient safety in simulation for mental health nursing education. Issues in mental health nursing. 2012;**33**(11):718-726. DOI: 10.3109/01612840.2012.709585

[56] Guinea S, Andersen P, Reid-Searl K, Levett-Jones T, Dwyer T, Heaton L, et al. Simulation-based learning for patient safety: The development of the Tag Team Patient Safety Simulation methodology for nursing education. Collegian. 2019;**26**(3):392-398. DOI: 10.1016/j.colegn.2018.09.008

[57] Joint Commission International. Available from: https://www.jointcommissioninternational.org/standards/international-patient-safety-goals/ [Accessed: 2020-07-28]

[58] National Patient Safety Foundation. Patient safety. 2016. Available from: http://www.npsf.org/?page=dictionarynz, [Accessed: 2020-07-28]

[59] Gurlek O, Kanber NA, Khorshid L. Investigating the use of identity wristbands in hospitals and patients' opinions/Hastanelerde kimlik tanimlayici bileklik kullanimina iliskin uygulamalarin ve hasta gorüslerinin incelenmesi. Journal of Education and Research in Nursing. 2015;**12**(3):195-204

[60] Henneman EA, Roche JP, Fisher DL, Cunningham H, Reilly CA, Nathanson BH, et al. Error identification and recovery by student nurses using human patient simulation: Opportunity to improve patient safety. Applied Nursing Research. 2010;**23**(1):11-21

[61] Bayram ŞB, Çalışkan N. Using a game-based virtual reality application in psychomotor skills acquisition: An experience sharing Oyun tabanlı sanal gerçeklik uygulamasının psikomotor beceri öğretiminde kullanımı: Bir deneyim paylaşımı. Journal of Human Sciences. 2019; 16(1), 155-163. DOI: 10.14687/jhs.v16i1.5508

[62] Biyik Bayram S. Effect of game based virtual reality application on tracheostomy care learning of nursing students, phd. thesis, Gazi University Institute of Health Sciences, december 2017

[63] Shibuy H, Eto C, Suzuki M, Imai R, Yamashita A, Nakano R, et al. Exploring the Possibility of Virtual Reality in Nursing Skills Education: A Preliminary Study Using a First-Person Video. Open Journal of Nursing. 2019;**9**(02):163. DOI: 10.4236/ojn.2019.92015

[64] Guise V, Chambers M, Välimäki M. What can virtual patient simulation offer mental health nursing education? Journal of psychiatric and mental health nursing. 2012;**19**(5):410-418. DOI: 10.1111/j.1365-2850.2011.01797.x

[65] Foronda CL, Swoboda SM, Hudson KW, Jones E, Sullivan N, Ockimey J, et al. Evaluation of vSIM for Nursing™: A trial of innovation. Clinical Simulation in Nursing. 2016;**12**(4):128-131. DOI: 10.1016/j.ecns.2015.12.006

[66] Liu T, Luo J, He H, Zheng J, Zhao J, Li K. History-taking instruction for baccalaureate nursing students by virtual patient training: A retrospective study. Nurse Education Today. 2018;**71**:97-104. DOI: 10.1016/j.nedt.2018.09.014

[67] Gu Y, Zou Z, Chen X. The effects of Vsim for nursing™ as a teaching strategy on fundamentals of nursing education in undergraduates. Clinical Simulation in Nursing. 2017;**13**(4):194-197. DOI: 10.1016/j.ecns.2017.01.005

[68] Luctkar-Flude M, Pulling C, Larocque M. Ending infusion confusion: evaluating a virtual intravenous pump educational module. Clinical Simulation in Nursing. 2012;**8**(2):39-48. DOI: 10.1016/j.ecns.2010.06.001

[69] Dubovi I, Levy ST, Dagan E. Now I know how! The learning process of medication administration among nursing students with non-immersive desktop virtual reality simulation. Computers & Education. 2017;**113**(16-27):16-27. DOI: 10.1016/j.compedu.2017.05.009

[70] Kruglikova I, Grantcharov TP, Drewes AM, Funch-Jensen P. Assessment of early learning curves among nurses and physicians using a high-fidelity virtual-reality colonoscopy simulator. Surgical Endoscopy. 2010;**24**(2):366-370. DOI: 10.1007/s00464-009-0555-7

[71] Weideman YL. Culleiton AL Innovation Center A Virtual Pregnancy for Pre-Licensure Nursing Students: Nine Months Up and Close. Nursing Education Perspectives. 2014;**35**(6):410-413. DOI: 10.5480/11-601.1

[72] Rice MM. Teams and teamwork in emergency medicine. Croskerry P, Cosby KS, Schenkel SM, Wears RL, editors. In: Patient safety in emergency medicine. 1st Ed., Philadelphia. Lippincott Williams & Wilkins, 2009;174-187p.

[73] Green J, Wyllie A, Jackson D. Virtual worlds: A new frontier for nurse education? Collegian. 2014;**21**(2):135-141. DOI: 10.1016/j.colegn.2013.11.004

[74] Uslusoy EÇ, Duran ET, Korkmaz M. safe injection practices. Hacettepe UniversitY Nursing Faculty Journal. 2016;**3**(2):50-57

[75] Potter PA, Perry AG. Fundamentals of nursing. (8th ed). St. Lous Missouri: Mosby Inc. 2013. 821-882p.

[76] Nakamura I, Fujita H, Tsukimori A, Kobayashi T, Sato A, Fukushima S, et al. Scenario-based simulation health care education for performance of hand hygiene. American journal of infection control. 2019;**47**(2):144-148. DOI: 10.1016/j.ajic.2018.07.024

[77] Farra SL, Smith S, Gillespie GL, Nicely S, Ulrich DL, Hodgson E, et al. Decontamination training: With and without virtual reality simulation. Advanced Emergency Nursing Journal. 2015;**37**(2):125-133. DOI: 10.1097/TME.0000000000000059

[78] Jung EY, Park DK, Lee YH, Jo HS, Lim YS, Park RW. Evaluation of practical exercises using an intravenous simulator incorporating virtual reality and haptics device technologies. Nurse Education Today. 2012;**32**(4):458-463. DOI: 10.1016/j.nedt.2011.05.012

[79] Engum SA, Jeffries P, Fisher L. Intravenous catheter training system: computer-based education versus traditional learning methods. The American Journal of Surgery. 2003;**186**(1):67-74. DOI: 10.1016/S0002-9610(03)00109-0

[80] Noyudom AN, Ketpichainarong W. Ruenwongsa, P. Development of a computer-based simulation unit on tracheal suctioning to enhance nursing students' knowledge and practical skills. The Thai Simulation 2011-TS'11-3rd Annual International Conference. 2011. Thailand.

[81] Bursiek AA, Hopkin MR, Breitkopf DM, Grubbs PL, Joswiak ME, Klipfel JM, et al. Use of high-fidelity simulation to enhance interdisciplinary collaboration and reduce patient falls. Journal of patient safety. 2020;**16**(3):245-250 www.journalpatientsafety.com

[82] DeBourgh GA, Prion SK. Using simulation to teach prelicensure nursing students to minimize patient risk and harm. Clinical Simulation in Nursing. 2011;7(2):47-56. DOI: 10.1016/j.ecns.2009.12.009

[83] Choi KS, He X, Chiang VCL, Deng Z. A virtual reality based simulator for learning nasogastric tube placement. Computers in Biology and Medicine. 2015;**57**:103-115. DOI: 10.1016/j.compbiomed.2014.12.006